THE BROCKPORT PHYSICAL FITNESS TRAINING GUIDE

Joseph P. Winnick, EdD

Francis X. Short, PED

State University of New York
College at Brockport

Editors

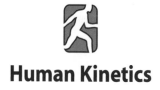

Human Kinetics

Library of Congress Cataloging-in-Publication Data

The Brockport physical fitness training guide / Joseph P. Winnick,
  Francis X. Short, editors.
     p.   cm.
  Includes bibliographical references (p.) and index.
  ISBN 0-7360-0120-4
  1. Physical fitness for children--Handbooks, manuals, etc.
  2. Exercise therapy for children--Handbooks, manuals, etc.
  3. Handicapped children--Development--Handbooks, manuals, etc.
  I. Winnick, Joseph P.   II. Short, Francis Xavier, 1950-   .
  RJ138.B76   1999   99-10379
  613.7'042--DC21   CIP

ISBN: 0-7360-0120-4

This book was developed as a part of Project Target which was conducted at the State University of New York, College at Brockport. Project Target was supported by the Office of Special Education and Rehabilitative Services (OSE/RS), U.S. Department of Education, Project No. HO23C30091. The contents presented herein are those of the authors and do not necessarily reflect the position or policy of OSE/RS or SUNY College at Brockport and no official endorsement should be inferred.

Acquisitions Editor: Michael S. Bahrke, PhD; **Developmental Editor:** Kristine Enderle; **Assistant Editor:** Amy Flaig; **Copyeditor:** Karen Slaght; **Indexer:** Sharon Duffy; **Graphic Designer:** Fred Starbird; **Graphic Artist:** Denise Lowry; **Cover Designer:** Jack Davis; **Photographers (interior):** Photo on pp. 22 and figure 3.1 on p. 48 by Dave Nishitani, all other photos provided by authors; **Illustrators:** Terry Hadyn, Mac illustrator; Tim Offenstein, line artist; **Printer:** United Graphics

Printed in the United States of America   10   9   8   7   6   5   4   3   2   1

Human Kinetics
Website: http://www.humankinetics.com/

United States: Human Kinetics, P.O. Box 5076, Champaign, IL 61825-5076
1-800-747-4457
e-mail: humank@hkusa.com

Canada: Human Kinetics, 475 Devonshire Road Unit 100, Windsor, ON N8Y 2L5
1-800-465-7301 (in Canada only)
e-mail: humank@hkcanada.com

Europe: Human Kinetics, P.O. Box IW14, Leeds LS16 6TR, United Kingdom
+44 (0)113-278 1708
e-mail: humank@hkeurope.com

Australia: Human Kinetics, 57A Price Avenue, Lower Mitcham, South Australia 5062
(08) 82771555
e-mail: humank@hkaustralia.com

New Zealand: Human Kinetics, P.O. Box 105-231, Auckland Central
09-523-3462
e-mail: humank@hknewz.com

CONTENTS

Chapter 4 Flexibility/Range of Motion   75
Paul Surburg

Annotated Resource List   121

Preface

Between 1993 and 1998, the Department of Education, Office of Special Education and Rehabilitative Services funded Project Target. The project was primarily designed to develop a criterion-referenced, health-related physical fitness test for youngsters with disabilities, ages 10 to 17. An educational component was included as a part of this project. This manual serves as part of the educational component. Specifically, it presents material to help develop the health-related physical fitness of youngsters with disabilities.

In developing this training manual, care was taken to coordinate it with the Brockport Physical Fitness Test (BPFT). Thus, terminology used is consistent with that used in the BPFT, and components of physical fitness and how they are measured are coordinated in both the test and training manuals developed as a part of Project Target. Standards for the evaluation and interpretation of health-related physical fitness are also coordinated. In essence, this training manual is designed to develop the physical fitness of youngsters with disabilities in association with results attained on the BPFT.

In chapter 1 of this manual, concepts important to training are covered. The chapter includes information dealing with health-related criterion-referenced testing, the interaction between physical activity and physical fitness, and the interaction between physical fitness and health. Individualized education programming, the lifetime commitment to physical activity and physical fitness, and safety precautions important to implementing programs are topics covered toward the end of the chapter.

Chapters 2, 3, and 4 relate to the development of components of physical fitness: cardiorespiratory endurance and body composition, muscular strength and endurance, and flexibility/range of motion. Each chapter presents information regarding the importance of components of physical fitness for health, how components of physical fitness are measured and evaluated in the BPFT, the underlying changes in the body affected by the development of physical fitness, factors influencing the development of physical fitness, and guidelines for developing and implementing physical fitness. Each chapter includes information related to the development of physical fitness of youngsters with disabilities.

There are several ways in which this manual is unique. First, it is special because it is the first of its kind designed to provide information regarding the development of the health-related physical fitness of children and adolescents with disabilities. The literature on this topic has emphasized guidelines for adults and/or for general populations. Another unique feature of this manual is that it recognizes and provides information that is designed to develop the functional as well as the physiological health of the individual. This is critical, as adequate physical fitness to conduct activities of daily living is crucial to persons with disabilities. A third unique feature of this manual is that it recommends guidelines for the development of physical fitness within the context of recommendations for physical activity provided by leading governmental and professional organizations. In this regard, the guidelines seek to develop health through physical activity, focusing upon the development of physical fitness. Finally, the manual is unique because suggested guidelines relate to general physical activity as well as to exercise, and they suggest modifications for persons with disabilities.

This book is designed to reach any qualified professional whose responsibility includes the health-related physical fitness development of youngsters with disabilities. However, the chief target group includes physical educators, both regular and adapted, and physical therapists working in educational settings.

It is our hope that this book provides a foundation for future development of this topic. Certainly much more will be learned in the future about health-related physical fitness as it relates to the needs and concerns of youngsters with disabilities. Appropriate training models for children; the relationship and interaction among health, physical activity, and physical fitness; and creative ways of motivating youngsters, parents, and professionals in realizing the importance of becoming involved with physical fitness programs are all areas rich with possibilities.

Acknowledgments

Writing this training manual was part of the educational component associated with Project Target. It was written to serve as a training component to be used in association with the Brockport Physical Fitness Test. Several persons helped the editors in its development, and it is important to recognize their contributions. First, thanks are extended to the invited professionals involved in writing the chapters. Each was invited because of their highly recognized expertise. Dr. Francis X. Short was the primary writer and editor of the second chapter following contributions to the chapter from Dr. Jeffrey McCubbin, Oregon State University and Dr. Georgia Frey, Texas A&M University. The third chapter was written by Dr. Patrick DiRocco, University of Wisconsin-LaCrosse, and the fourth chapter was written by Dr. Paul Surburg, Indiana University. Dr. Joseph P. Winnick served as primary editor of these chapters and worked closely with these authors in developing guidelines for training and encouraging a health-related perspective.

In developing a training manual, the creation of figures is an important task. Thanks are sincerely extended to the many persons who served as subjects in photos. In particular, David Maxwell must be thanked for his cheerful willingness to help. Thanks are also extended to James Dusen, Photographic Services at SUNY Brockport, and Pam Maryjanowski, Empire State Games for the Physically Challenged, for their help with photographs. Finally, thanks are extended to Melissa Zurlo for her work in typing this manuscript repeatedly and Lori Erickson, graduate assistant associated with Project Target, for several contributions important in developing this training manual.

1

INTRODUCTION

Joseph P. Winnick

This book is designed to provide basic information needed to develop health-related physical fitness in youngsters with disabilities. The target audience is teachers and program leaders who are responsible for developing physical fitness. The book has been designed as an educational component associated with the Brockport Physical Fitness Test (BPFT)—a health-related criterion-referenced physical fitness test that can be used to identify the health-related physical fitness status and unique needs of youngsters. Although it was designed to be used with the BPFT, this book can be used separately as a resource for guidelines for the development of health-related physical fitness. The chapters cover the development of cardiorespiratory endurance (CRE) and body composition (BC), muscular strength and endurance, and flexibility/range of motion (ROM). After reading this book, teachers and program leaders should know how to develop physical fitness. Although many suggested activities for the development of physical fitness are provided in the book, emphasis is placed on the principles and guidelines that underlie activity selection. Information on additional activities is available in other sources, some of which are provided in the appendix included at the end of the book.

BRIEF BACKGROUND OF HEALTH-RELATED CRITERION-REFERENCED PHYSICAL FITNESS TESTING

The development of physical fitness in school-aged youngsters in the United States has received considerable attention since data presented by Kraus and Hirschland (1954) indicated that American youngsters were less fit than their European counterparts. Partly in response to this study, there emerged an interest in the development of tests of physical fitness. Notable among these was the American Association for Health, Physical Education, and Recreation (AAHPER) Youth Fitness Test published in 1958 and revised in subsequent years. In the 1970s, an interest emerged in developing a physical fitness test designed to measure health-related physical fitness, and the American Alliance for Health, Physical Education, Recreation and Dance (AAHPERD) published its first health-related test in 1980. As tests of health-related physical fitness were being conceptualized and published, criterion-referenced standards were increasingly used for the evaluation of health-related physical fitness. This change was inevitable, as criteria for evaluation inherently needed to change from comparisons of performance with others to comparisons to indices of health status. In the 1980s and 1990s, interest in and use of health-related physical fitness tests has increased, with more and more evidence supporting the importance of both physical fitness and physical activity for health benefits (Blair, 1993; Bouchard, Shephard, and Stephens, 1994; Consensus Development Conference, 1995; Pate et al. 1995; Paffenbarger and Lee, 1996). In 1996, AAHPERD endorsed the Prudential *FITNESSGRAM* (Cooper Institute of Aerobics Research [CIAR], 1992) as its recommended test of health-related criterion-referenced physical fitness for persons, ages 5 to 17.

Although attention was given to the development of health-related physical fitness tests for nondisabled youngsters in the 1990s, no comprehensive health-related criterion-referenced tests had been designed for use with youngsters with disabilities. In response to this situation, the U.S. Department of Education, Office of Special Education and Rehabilitation Services, funded Project Target between 1993 and 1998. This research project was conducted at the State University of New York, College at Brockport under the leadership of Joseph P. Winnick and Francis X. Short. It was designed to establish and validate a health-related criterion-referenced test for youths with disabilities, ages 10 to 17. The work served as a basis for the development of the BPFT (Winnick and Short, 1999). Components and test items for the BPFT appear in table 1.1. Although 27 test items are listed, only four to six items are typically selected for each youngster tested. Criterion-referenced standards are provided with each test item and serve as a basis for the assessment of health-related physical fitness. This training manual has been designed to improve health-related physical fitness in association with the BPFT.

PHYSICAL ACTIVITY AND PHYSICAL FITNESS

Bouchard and Shephard (1994) define physical activity as any bodily movement produced by skeletal muscle resulting in a substantial increase over resting energy expenditure. Caspersen, Powell, and Christenson (1985) define physical fitness as a set of attributes that people have or achieve that relate to the ability to perform physical activity. For the purposes of this training program, health-related physical fitness refers to those components of fitness that are affected by habitual physical activity and relate to health status. It is defined as a state characterized by (a) an ability to perform and sustain daily activities and (b) the demonstration of traits or capacities that are associated with a low risk of premature development of diseases and conditions related to movement (adapted from Pate, 1988).

The relationship among health, physical activity, and health-related physical fitness for the BPFT and this training manual is represented by the conceptual model presented in figure 1.1. As shown, physical activity provides a continuing benefit for the development of physical fitness, which in turn contributes to health. Frequency, intensity, and duration define patterns of physical activity. These can be manipulated to most efficiently and effectively develop desired levels of the components of health-related physical fitness. Ways to enhance fitness are included

Table 1.1   Components and Test Items for the Brockport Physical Fitness Test (BPFT)

Aerobic function
20-m PACER
Modified 16-m PACER
Target aerobic movement test (TAMT)
One-mile run/walk

Body composition
Skinfold measures
Body mass index (BMI)

Musculoskeletal function	
Muscular strength and endurance	**Flexibility or range of motion**
Bench press	Modified Apley test
Curl-up	Back-saver sit and reach
Modified curl-up	Shoulder stretch
Dumbbell press	Modified Thomas test
Extended arm hang	Target stretch test (TST)
Flexed arm hang	
Dominant grip strength	
Isometric push-up	
Pull-up	
Modified pull-up	
Push-up	
40-m push/walk	
Reverse curl	
Seated push-up	
Trunk lift	
Wheelchair ramp test	

in guidelines presented with the development of physical fitness in later chapters. The health-related components of physical fitness to be addressed in chapters.

The model also depicts the relationship between physical activity and health. Physical activity for health is highly accepted and is currently widely advocated. The 1996 Surgeon General's Report (U.S. Department of Health and Human Services, 1996) on physical activity and health states that significant health benefits

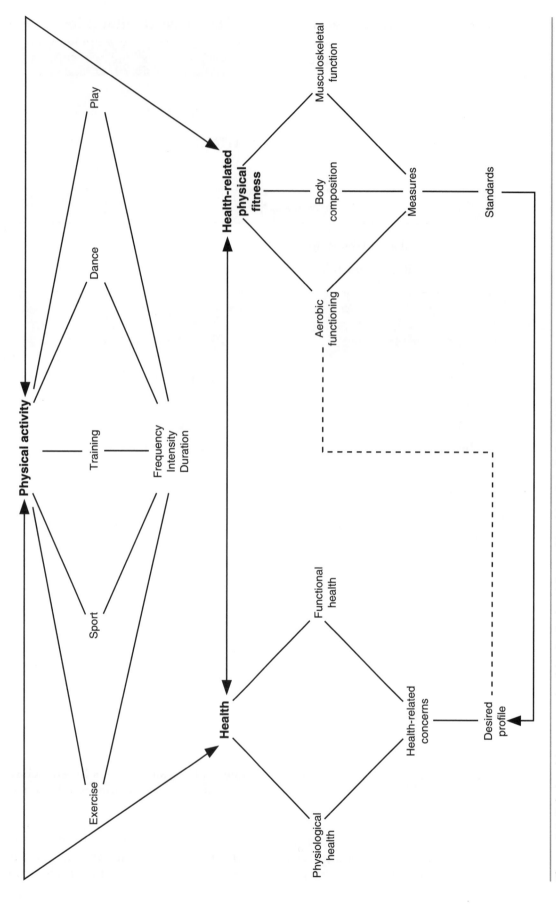

Figure 1.1 Relationships among health, physical activity, and health-related physical fitness

can be attained by engaging in moderate physical activity (e.g., 30 minutes of brisk walking) on most, if not all, days of the week. The report also acknowledges that for most people, greater health benefits can be obtained by engaging in physical activity more vigorously or longer. The American College of Sports Medicine (ACSM), the Centers for Disease Control and Prevention (CDC) (Pate et al., 1995), and the President's Council on Physical Fitness and Sports (PCPFS) (1996) agree with this position and recommend that Americans accumulate at least 30 minutes of moderate-intensity physical activity on most, preferably all, days of the week. This is sometimes referred to as the lifetime physical activity guideline (Pangrazzi, Corbin, and Welk, 1996, p. 39). The 1992 Second International Consensus Symposium on Physical Activity, Fitness, and Health published a consensus statement indicating support for 30 to 60 minutes of physical activity nearly every day and, in addition, a recommendation that adolescents engage in three or more sessions per week of activities that last 20 minutes or more and require moderate to vigorous levels of exertion (Bouchard, Shephard, and Stephens, 1994).

In 1998, the Council for Physical Education for Children (COPEC, n.d.) published a statement of guidelines indicating that on all or most days of the week, elementary-school-aged children (ages 5 to 12) should accumulate at least 30 to 60 minutes of physical activity that is age- and developmentally appropriate. The guidelines recommend 10 to 15 minutes or more of moderate to vigorous activity each day. However, the guidelines encourage an accumulation of more than 60 minutes and up to several hours per day of appropriate activity for elementary-school-aged children.

Involvement in physical activity and the development of physical fitness go hand in hand, and each can contribute to health status. For the purpose of this manual, emphasis is placed on recommended patterns of physical activity (as defined by frequency, intensity, and duration) designed to enhance specific components of health-related physical fitness. Where appropriate, however, these patterns also will be consistent with the current physical activity recommendations for enhancing health status discussed in the previous paragraphs. The guidelines that appear in subsequent chapters will relate to both exercise and general activity experiences for the development of physical fitness for the general population and, as needed, modifications for youths with disabilities. The physical activity guidelines presented above pertain to the general population and may be modified for individuals with disabilities in accord with an individualized education program (IEP).

HEALTH-RELATED PHYSICAL FITNESS AND HEALTH

The model depicted in figure 1.1 also conveys a relationship between health-related physical fitness and health. As stated earlier, much attention has recently been given to identifying the health benefits of physical activity and physical fitness. The Prudential *FITNESSGRAM* (CIAR, 1992) is a test of health-related physical fitness focusing on the general population. It indicates that acceptable levels of aerobic capacity are associated with a reduced risk of high blood pressure, coronary heart disease, obesity, diabetes, some forms of cancer, and other health problems in adults. Acceptable levels of percentage body fat are associated with reducing risk factors associated with heart disease, and acceptable levels of musculoskeletal functioning are important in maintaining functional health and correct posture, thereby reducing possibilities of future lower back pain and restrictions in independent living.

The BPFT was developed with the assumption that youngsters with disabilities typically have the same health-related concerns associated with a lack of physical activity and fitness as their nondisabled peers. However, they also have additional specific health-related concerns that may relate to fitness. These health-related needs may encompass physiological and/or functional health. Youngsters with disabilities may need to give particular attention to health-related needs associated with the ability to sustain aerobic behavior, perform activities of independent living, lift and transfer the body from a wheelchair, propel a wheelchair, maintain muscular balance and body symmetry, overcome architectural barriers, develop functional and/or optimal levels of flexibility/ROM, and maintain appropriate BC. The BPFT recognizes the uniqueness of health needs of youngsters with disabilities and applies this notion to the development of a personalized process of developing a health-related physical fitness test for the measurement and evaluation of health-related physical fitness. More detailed information on the conceptual model presented in figure 1.1 may be found in the BPFT test manual (Winnick and Short, 1999).

INDIVIDUALIZED EDUCATION PROGRAMS AND THE DEVELOPMENT OF HEALTH-RELATED PHYSICAL FITNESS

The Individuals with Disabilities Education Act (IDEA) has been designed to assure that all children with disabilities have available to them special education and related services designed to meet their unique needs. Furthermore, it clearly states that special education means specially designed instruction, including instruction in physical education. Rules and regulations associated with IDEA include the development of physical fitness as a part of the definition of physical education.

IDEA requires that every child receiving special education have an IEP and that physical education be included. In cases where a child has a unique physical education need and a specially designed program is appropriate, physical education would be included in all components of the IEP.

The health-related physical fitness of an individual should be a key element in a quality physical education program. As a health-related criterion-referenced test of physical fitness, the BPFT may be used to identify the present level of performance, identify unique needs, and establish annual goals including short-term objectives. An important step in assuring acceptable physical fitness levels is to determine a youngster's present level of performance. This information helps determine if the youngster has a unique physical education need for the basis of an annual goal and to help identify a starting point for physical fitness development.

Youngsters who don't meet minimally acceptable levels of health-related physical fitness exhibit a unique need that can serve as a basis for an identified annual goal. For example, if a youngster fails to successfully complete the target aerobic movement test (TAMT) requiring 15 minutes of continuous moderate physical activity and that standard is the minimally acceptable level of aerobic behavior appropriate for the youngster, a unique need in the area of aerobic behavior is exhibited. An appropriate annual goal for this youngster is to develop aerobic behavior. As the TAMT is administered, program leaders can gain information to establish reasonable short-term objectives. For example, if the youngster was able to continue moderate physical activity for 10 minutes, this is a measure of present level of performance that is attained and is a level from which a short-term objective can be set. For example, if 10 minutes is the present level of performance, a short-term objective may be 11 or 12 minutes and the attainment of the annual goal, of course, would be 15 minutes (representing a minimal acceptable level of aerobic behavior).

When administering the BPFT, scores representing student performance will be attained and then used in determining whether health-related standards are met. As performance is reviewed and interpreted, strengths and weaknesses of a youngster can be objectively identified. Based on information collected, an individualized profile can be established for each youngster. In developing a profile, a subjective appraisal to account for test results can also be developed. For example, test results may be influenced by factors such as condition of a wheelchair, time of day, cooperation, and learning. The results of subjective appraisal should be noted and used, as judgments are made in regard to an IEP.

Schools and agencies should develop and follow written plans for IEP development. Not reaching minimally acceptable health-related criterion-referenced standards considered appropriate for a youngster in one or more component areas of physical fitness, for example, can serve as a basis for the identification of unique need(s). Goals, which are generic statements designed to give direction to instructional or developmental programs, can be identified from this information. Table 1.2 provides sample entries in three parts of an IEP for a male, age 14, with mental retardation (MR) and mild limitations in physical fitness based on administration

Table 1.2   Sample Entries in an Individualized Education Program (IEP)

Gender: Male   Age: 14   Classification: Mental retardation with mild limitations in physical fitness
Present level of performance:
The student sustains moderate physical activity for 10 min on the TAMT (fails to meet general standard).
The sum of triceps and subscapular skinfolds is 22 mm (meets preferred general standard).
The student reaches 8 in. on the back-saver sit and reach (meets general standard).
The student attains a score of 9 in. on the trunk lift (meets general standard).
The student receives a score of 25 kg on the dominant grip strength test (meets specific standard; fails to meet minimal general standard).
The student performs a flexed arm hang for 6 s (unable to meet specific standard).
The student performs 16 modified curl-ups (meets specific standard; fails to meet minimal general standard).
Annual goal(s):
The student will increase upper body strength and endurance.
The student will increase aerobic behavior.
Short-term objective(s):
The student will perform a flexed arm hang for 8 s (represents specific standard).
The student will sustain moderate physical activity for 15 min on the TAMT (meets general standard).

of the BPFT. In addition to typically reported information, several of the entries in table 1.2 give information related to standards associated with the BPFT. Specific standards are measures of attainment associated with a defined category of persons and/or are standards that are adjusted for the effects of impairment or disability. General standards are measures of attainment associated with the general population and may be appropriate for youngsters with a disability. A general standard is not adjusted for the effects of impairment or disability. A minimal general standard is the lowest acceptable health-related criterion-referenced level of attainment for the general population, and a single or preferred standard is a good health-related criterion-referenced level of attainment for the general population. (While criteria for determining the presence of a unique need should be established locally, comparisons to general, rather than specific, standards for this purpose usually are most appropriate.)

In an IEP, information pertaining to present level of performance and short-term objectives is provided. A program leader must decide how great a change can and should be made in each circumstance. Setting short-term objectives in consideration of acceptable standards is a recommended procedure.

Once the present level of performance is determined, annual goals are established, and short-term instructional objectives are set, program leaders should identify appropriate physical activity and exercise recommendations for and/or with the youngster(s). As activities are selected and provided, choose progressions or exercise prescriptions to enhance development of physical fitness. Individualized education programs applying guidelines for physical fitness development will most efficiently and effectively move the youngster from the present level of performance to short-term instructional objectives. Guidelines for the development of CRE, appropriate BC, muscular strength and endurance, and ROM/ flexibility are presented in subsequent chapters of this book to help program leaders plan and implement programs.

The settings in which to implement programs must be decided on and arranged. In schools, roles and responsibilities of physical education teachers, therapists, and classroom teachers should be identified. Decisions should be made in regard to time given to formalized exercise-oriented programs and diverse broad-based physical education offerings. The willingness to participate in enjoyed activities is a key concept that should be emphasized for the development and maintenance of health-related physical fitness and for a lifetime commitment to physical activity. However, it may also be important to help youngsters reach minimal levels of health-related physical fitness through exercise. Although perhaps not as enjoyable, exercises may be necessary for the health of the individual.

A LIFETIME COMMITMENT TO PHYSICAL ACTIVITY AND PHYSICAL FITNESS

Although the development of health-related physical fitness is an important goal in school programs, including IEPs for youngsters with disabilities, it is important to realize that involvement in developing physical activity experiences throughout the total life span is the single most important goal of health-related physical fitness programs. Regular physical activity contributes to physical fitness, and physical fitness, in turn, enhances involvement in quality physical activity experiences. Benefits in health are gained from desirable levels of physical activity and physical fitness. To receive these gains, persons need to reach and maintain recommended levels of physical activity involvement and acceptable levels of physical fitness.

An individual is most likely to engage in lifetime physical activity if the activity is fun and brings pleasure. Especially for children, this means involvement in physical activity during play, dynamic physical education experiences, recreation, or other active experiences. Although goals and objectives related to physical fitness should be included as important parts of IEPs, the activities to develop these should be enjoyable, developmentally appropriate, and offered in an appropriate setting by a stimulating teacher. Although exercises may be critically important and should be employed as needed, physical activity programs must be broader in scope than simply providing calisthenics or exercises. Whenever possible, activities that are enjoyable to the participant should be used for physical fitness objectives. For example, reaching for a stimulating balloon extended overhead is more fun than responding to a cue to lift the arm upward toward the sky as part of a calisthenic routine. Horseback riding is probably more fun for kids with cerebral palsy (CP) needing to increase lower limb ROM than typical exercises are.

The development of physical fitness and lifetime involvement is enhanced by programs that are broad in scope. Again, rather than restricting participation to formal exercise programs, it is important to introduce and involve youngsters in many different activities. From exposure to and the development of skills in a variety of activities, an individual is more likely to find an activity enjoyed throughout the life span. As persons engage in enjoyable activities, they develop skills to a higher level, which in turn, brings satisfaction and greater involvement. Teaching skills for successful participation, thus, becomes a key dimension for lifetime involvement in health-related physical activity and fitness (see figure 1.2).

Consideration was given to success in developing standards associated with the BPFT. Test developers selected items in the test that youngsters could learn and perform and standards that were both health-related and attainable. These considerations were seen as important because youngsters need a reasonable chance of success as they strive to attain health-related standards.

Several recognition and awards programs have been effectively employed to motivate youngsters to attain higher levels of performance and participation in

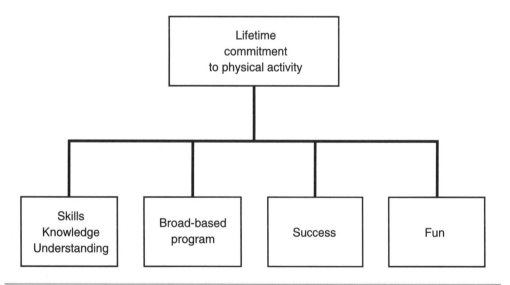

Figure 1.2 Key features for a lifetime commitment to physical activity

physical activity (Prudential *FITNESSGRAM*, PCPFS, AAHPERD). Recently developed recognition and awards programs recognize both behavior and performance. Completion of exercise logs, achievement of specific goals, and fulfillment of contractual agreements are examples of how desirable behavior can be recognized. Successful achievement or improvement related to health-related fitness also can be recognized. An important point to be made is that some system should be designed to motivate youngsters to pursue physical activity and desirable levels of health-related physical fitness. It is particularly important to youngsters with disabilities to have the same recognition and awards available for those with and without disabilities and to have provisions to permit equal opportunity to attain recognition and awards. This may require adjustments in test items, standards, and procedures for persons with disabilities that are equivalent to rather than identical to those of their nondisabled peers. Pangrazzi and Corbin (1994) provide an example of how a recognition program may be modified as they suggest ways of applying the Prudential *FITNESSGRAM* recognition program for students.

Programs designed to prepare youngsters for a lifetime commitment to physical activity and physical fitness should include knowledge and understanding about health-related physical activity and physical fitness in their programs. The importance of physical activity and fitness to health should be the basis of such a program. Youngsters would benefit from knowledge and understanding of the meaning of physical fitness and its components, guidelines for developing it, how it may be assessed, how to conduct self-assessment, how to establish objectives and goals, and other concepts on how to engage in safe and effective programs. They would also benefit from knowledge and understanding of the benefits of physical activity to health; the value of various types of activity; concepts related to intensity, frequency, and duration of activity; how to effectively incorporate physical activity into their lifestyle; and developing and keeping activity logs.

GENERAL SAFETY PRECAUTIONS IN DEVELOPING PHYSICAL FITNESS

In the chapters that follow, many specific safety precautions related to the development of physical fitness will be presented. Several general safety precautions, however, are presented here.

• Physical fitness programs for individuals with disabilities should be supervised and directly implemented by qualified personnel. Appropriate standards for qualification should be met by teachers or other professionals providing direct services.

• Youngsters, parents, professionals, and other service providers must understand that there is no way to completely eliminate the risk of injury during exercise testing or participation. However, the overall absolute risk in the general population is low, especially when weighed against the health benefits of exercise (ACSM, 1995).

• The information presented in this book regarding implementation of programs designed to develop physical fitness is given with the assumption that physical activity has been deemed appropriate for each youngster and/or that physical activity is provided in accord with parameters specified by competent personnel.

• Physical activity may need to be terminated if youngsters experience dizziness or appear to be in extreme discomfort or pain.

• Progressions in the frequency, intensity, and duration of activity should follow recommended practices. Initial levels of activity should not be overly aggressive and should consider muscle soreness, discomfort, and injury.

• A survey of medical history and a physical examination are important in starting and implementing an exercise program. Underlying causes of disability, injuries secondary to disability, and medication are factors that need to be considered in establishing appropriate physical activity involvement (Lockette and Keyes, 1994).

2

Cardiorespiratory Endurance and Body Composition

Francis X. Short, Jeffrey McCubbin, & Georgia Frey

This chapter presents guidelines for the development of cardiorespiratory endurance (CRE) and body composition (BC) for youths with disabilities, ages 10 to 17. In certain parts of the chapter information relating to CRE and BC is separated, and in other parts it is included under a combined heading. The chapter defines, presents benefits of, identifies biological aspects related to, suggests ways of measuring, discusses general factors influencing, and presents guidelines for developing CRE and appropriate levels of BC. Particular attention is given to the development associated with individuals with disabilities.

CARDIORESPIRATORY ENDURANCE, BODY COMPOSITION, AND HEALTH

During the 1990s much attention has been given to identifying and analyzing the benefits of physical activity for health. For example, a comprehensive review was presented in the first Surgeon General's Report on physical activity and health (U.S. Department of Health and Human Services, 1996). In table 2.1, health benefits from physical activity based on this report are presented in categories that relate to this chapter. Table 2.1 makes it obvious that physical activity, in general, and specific activities to enhance the development of CRE and appropriate BC, in particular, are of significant importance to the health of the human.

Although important for all, numerous subgroups of the population are particularly at risk for not being physically active on a regular basis. These groups include women, people of lower socioeconomic status, selected racial/ethnic groups, and people with disabilities. It is imperative that teachers, parents, and health care professionals work with all individuals, and particularly with populations that are at risk of being inactive, to become more physically active on a regular

Table 2.1   Some Health Benefits from Physical Activity

Cardiovascular health
Decreases risk of cardiovascular disease mortality
Prevents or delays development of high blood pressure
Prevents or reduces the severity of atherosclerosis
Increases coronary blood flow
Improves efficiency of oxygen exchange
Increases high density lipids (HDL)
Obesity and weight control
Enhances weight control
Improves appearance
Affects distribution of body fat favorably
Reduces blood fat
Other areas
Decreases risk of colon cancer
Lowers risk of noninsulin dependent diabetes mellitus
Enhances achieving and maintaining peak bone mass
Improves ability to perform activities of daily living
Reduces risk of falling
Reduces symptoms of depression and anxiety

Source: U.S. Department of Health and Human Services: Effects of Physical Activity on Health and Disease: Surgeon General's Report on Physical Activity and Health, 1996.

basis. This may include participation in structured exercise-based programs and/ or involvement in a variety of enjoyed physical activities. The long-term effects of inactivity by persons with disabilities has become a major issue for the public health community. For example, persons with spinal cord injuries (SCIs) are at greater risk for myocardial infarction than the general population. Individuals with disabilities, in general, are at greater risk for obesity, which in turn increases the risk of death prior to age 65 (Heath and Fentem, 1997).

Inactivity may be as great a risk factor for coronary heart disease in the general population as hypertension, high cholesterol, and smoking (Heath and Fentem, 1997). Inactivity, however, is a greater threat to people with disabilities because the disability itself may prohibit or limit activity (see figure 2.1). Youngsters with physical impairments, for instance, may not have access to formal activity programs, may be restricted in the kinds of activities they can do, or may be discouraged from participating. Similarly, youngsters with visual impairments may be

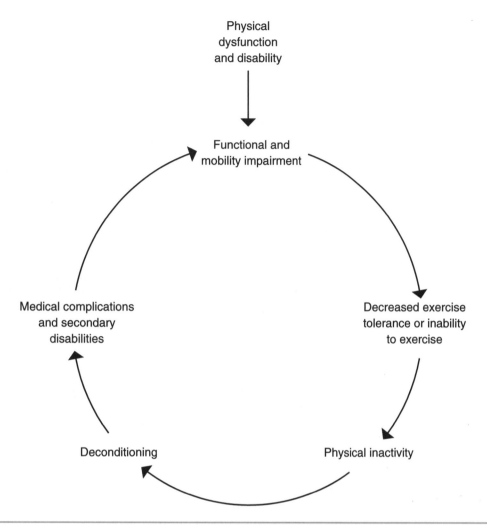

Figure 2.1 The cycle of disability, inactivity, and functional decline
Reprinted with permission from Miller, P. (1995). *Fitness Programming and Physical Disability*. Champaign, IL: Human Kinetics, p. 52.

overprotected or may not receive the necessary accommodations (partners, guide wires, adapted equipment, etc.) to participate, whereas youngsters with mental retardation (MR) may not be intrinsically motivated to participate or know how to locate community-based activity programs. Bringing attention to the long-term implications of physical inactivity in these populations is a major challenge.

Rimmer (1994), following an extensive review of the literature, reports that childhood and adolescent obesity is prevalent (approximately 20% of children are obese), is on the rise (at least a 39% increase since the mid-1960s), is a significant health problem (obese children are at greater risk for respiratory impairments, diabetes, orthopedic disorders, and psychological dysfunction), and is associated with obesity in adults (40 to 70% of obese children grow to be obese adults). Obesity in adults has been linked to a number of health-related problems including coronary heart disease, diabetes, colon cancer, hypertension, and musculoskeletal disorders. Obesity predisposes the individual not only to an increased risk of certain diseases but also to reduced functional ability resulting from impaired work efficiency and an increased risk of injury from chronic stress. A "vicious cycle" can evolve whereby obesity contributes to inactivity, which, in turn, reinforces obesity.

The basic cause of obesity is an imbalance between the intake of food and daily energy expenditure (Shephard, 1994). Youngsters with disabilities are at particular risk for obesity because their daily energy expenditure is often reduced as a result of the disability. Youngsters with disabilities, in general, tend to be less active than their nondisabled counterparts. They may be stimulated less to move, find movement to be more difficult, and find places in which to move to be less accessible. Youngsters who must use wheelchairs for mobility purposes typically burn even fewer calories during physical activity because movement is conducted with a smaller muscle mass ("arms-only" activity versus "whole-body" activity). It is not surprising, therefore, that research studies have found significantly larger skinfold values for children and adolescents with MR (Rarick, Dobbins, and Broadhead, 1976; Rarick and McQuillan, 1977) and for those with visual impairments, spinal neuromuscular conditions, and congenital anomalies or amputations (Winnick and Short, 1982) when compared to nondisabled controls. Some youngsters with cerebral palsy (CP), however, provide an "exception to the rule." Hypertonic muscles and mechanical inefficiency frequently associated with CP may result in higher daily energy expenditures and yield skinfold values that are either similar to or smaller than those obtained by nondisabled peers.

For youngsters with disabilities, it is essential for parents and teachers to understand that inactivity may have long-term health implications complicated by obesity. The risk factors associated with hypokinetic disease develop very early in life and are not just considerations for adult fitness programs. As an example, for persons with MR it is critically important that healthy eating habits and physical activity are reinforced by teachers and peer models. Obesity is not a disorder that is easily treated, yet it can be prevented with appropriate physical activity and diet patterns started during childhood and adolescence.

CARDIORESPIRATORY ENDURANCE

In this context, cardiorespiratory endurance is defined as the ability to perform large muscle, dynamic, moderate- to high- intensity exercise for prolonged periods (American College of Sports Medicine [ACSM], 1995). It is a component of health-related physical fitness that depends on the state of the cardiovascular, respiratory, and skeletal muscle systems. Associated factors include submaximal exercise capacity, maximal aerobic power, heart functions, lung functions, and blood pressure (Bouchard and Shephard, 1994). CRE relates to the ability of the body to use oxygen to produce energy. In relation to the Brockport Physical Fitness Test (BPFT), the term *aerobic functioning* is interchangeable with the term *cardiorespiratory endurance*. For purposes of measurement, aerobic functioning in the BPFT includes two components: aerobic behavior and aerobic capacity. Aerobic behavior relates to the ability to sustain physical activity of a specific intensity for a particular duration. Aerobic capacity relates to the highest rate of oxygen that can be consumed by a person while exercising.

The Measurement of Aerobic Functioning in the Brockport Physical Fitness Test (BPFT)

The target aerobic movement test (TAMT) is the test item used to measure aerobic behavior in the BPFT. Level I of the test measures the ability of students to sustain moderate physical activity for 15 minutes. Levels II and III of the test may be used to measure the ability to sustain low-level vigorous or vigorous activity, respectively. The type of physical activity to elicit an elevated heart rate (HR) can take any form desired as long as the target HR intensity is maintained. Examples include jogging, wheeling, dancing, walking, running, performing aerobics, and playing tag.

Aerobic capacity refers to the highest rate of oxygen that can be consumed by a person while exercising. In the BPFT, this is estimated by the Progressive Aerobic Cardiovascular Endurance Run (PACER) test and the one-mile run/walk test. The PACER test measures the ability to complete laps marked out at either 16 or 20 meters within a prescribed time period. The time interval for laps gets progressively shorter as the test proceeds, requiring increased running speed as the test continues. The 16-m PACER is used for students with MR and mild limitations in physical fitness. In the one-mile run/walk, participants complete one mile in the fastest possible time period. Time to complete the run/walk is recorded. The BPFT allows for partners to be used if the student is blind.

Basic Understanding of the Cardiorespiratory System

The basic elements of the cardiorespiratory system include the heart, lungs, and peripheral tissues that supply oxygen to working muscles. The ability of our bodies to use oxygen during exercise depends on the ability of the systems to take in, transport, and utilize available oxygen (Figoni, 1995). Any conditions that negatively affect the function of these systems reduce the ability to use oxygen and limit functional aerobic capacity.

Aerobic exercise involves sustaining an elevated HR over a long period of time. This typically requires a person to use a continuous form of exercise, with large muscle groups working repetitively over time to stress the system. Aerobic or cardiorespiratory training relies on stressing the systems that provide oxygen to the working muscles. Adaptations by the cardiorespiratory system due to training occur after the system has been stressed beyond its normal working capacity. This positive form of stress causes adaptations resulting in more efficient heart and lung functions. The primary stimulus for more efficient heart function is an increased workload proportional to the size of muscle mass activity involved in exercise. Thus, persons with larger muscle mass can accommodate greater amounts of stress than those with less muscle mass (e.g., people with SCI).

The heart's ability to pump blood to the circulatory system is referred to as cardiac output. Cardiac output is represented by stroke volume × heart rate. Stroke volume is the amount of blood ejected from the left ventricle of the heart with each contraction. The more blood flowing into the heart, the greater potential for increasing stroke volume. An efficient, trained heart has the capacity for a greater stroke volume and thus can reduce the frequency of HR response to the same exercise intensity. Persons with paralyzed or inactive limbs will likely have a reduced capacity to have blood flow return to the heart and thus have a lower potential for stroke volume.

If exercise intensity increases and stroke volume is not changed, two other responses will occur. HR response will reach a maximal level more quickly, and/or energy sources will be insufficient, causing fatigue and reducing the person's ability to maintain exercise at a given intensity. HR response is under the control of the autonomic nervous system. Disruption of normal autonomic nervous system response can negatively affect the HR response to exercise and limit a person's aerobic capacity.

Physiologic Systems That Support Aerobic Exercise

There are three primary systems that support aerobic exercise: (1) oxygen intake and pulmonary ventilation, (2) oxygen transport and circulation, and (3) oxygen utilization and aerobic metabolism. Each of these systems may be affected by a disabling condition, yet all also have the capacity to respond positively to training.

The pulmonary system contains the lungs, airways, and musculature to support ventilation. Oxygen enters the system and is perfused through the vessels to eventually deliver oxygen to working muscles. Carbon dioxide and other waste products are diffused through venous circulation and exhaled back into the atmosphere. Pulmonary ventilation can be affected by asthma, pulmonary diseases, and high-level SCI that affect inspiratory musculature. Polio, muscular dystrophies, or, in some cases, multiple sclerosis (MS) can affect ventilatory musculature, limiting inspiration or expiration.

The oxygen transport system maintains the flow of oxygen and nutrients to the exercising muscles. Normally the central circulatory system (heart and pulmonary system) channels blood via the arterial system to supply energy to the muscles and returns waste products, including carbon dioxide, via the venous system. Sympathetic input from the autonomic nervous system regulates blood flow and cardiac output. In addition, the autonomic nervous system affects vasodilation and vasoconstriction of the vascular system to insure that muscles receive nutrients when exercising. Disabilities that affect the autonomic nervous system can impair overall effectiveness of oxygen transport. Examples include high-level SCI (above T4), MS, and neuromuscular diseases. Exercise hypotension, or low blood pressure, can occur in high-level SCI. This negatively affects the body's ability to shunt oxygen-depleted blood back to the heart for re-oxygenation. This, in combination with muscular paralysis, leads to venous pooling limiting exercise tolerance. Several techniques may help with this problem. These include using a more horizontal position while exercising, using compressive abdominal binders and support hose, and increasing fluid intake (Figoni, 1995). Some disabilities that include hypertonicity, such as spastic CP, may actually occlude blood flow, also limiting the ability of the body to perform aerobic work.

Oxygen is utilized or metabolized by skeletal muscle to support physical activity. There are two types of metabolism—anaerobic and aerobic. Anaerobic metabolism takes place in the absence of oxygen and is a relatively rapid but limited energy source. Anaerobic activities are conducted at near maximal effort and typically last for less than three minutes. Aerobic metabolism, on the other hand, combines oxygen with food fuels to produce more energy per molecule of glucose than does anaerobic metabolism and can potentially support activity for longer periods. Aerobic activities are those that are submaximal and performed for a prolonged period of time. When the energy demands of the activity do not exceed the ability of the body to utilize oxygen, the individual is said to be exercising at a steady state. However, when the energy demands (intensity) of the activity surpass the body's ability to utilize oxygen, the activity will be performed anaerobically, and the duration of the activity will diminish due to fatigue. Oxygen utilization can be affected by disability if there is a reduced exercising muscle mass (e.g., propelling wheelchairs with arms rather than running with legs), impaired coordination of muscle action (e.g., incoordination due to CP), or general deconditioning (e.g., muscular weakness and inefficiency due to an inactive lifestyle).

Cardiorespiratory Training

The desired goal of improving cardiorespiratory function is to positively impact the overall health of the participant. As already mentioned, certain levels of CRE have been shown to reduce the risk in adults of certain diseases, including hypertension, coronary heart disease, obesity, diabetes, and some forms of cancer (Cureton, 1994). Also, the ability to sustain aerobic activity has relevance for the performance of daily activities and is considered to be an indication of one's "functional health." If training programs are established at the appropriate intensity, frequency, and duration, most individuals will be able to develop their CRE and enjoy better physiological and functional health.

Manipulating the variables of intensity (how hard?), frequency (how often?), and duration (how long?) of activity is critical to the success of a CRE training program. Instructors should recognize that these variables are interrelated so that changes in one may appropriately result in changes in another. For instance, one activity program that is more intense but of a shorter duration may convey similar health benefits to another activity program that is less intense but of longer duration.

Quantifying appropriate levels of frequency and duration is fairly straightforward. Frequency generally is expressed in terms of the number of days in a week that activity is performed (e.g., three to five days per week, two times a day, five to seven days per week, etc.). Duration is simply monitored by timing the length of the activity period (e.g., 20 minutes, 60 minutes, etc.). Tracking intensity, particularly in a field setting, however, is somewhat less objective and a bit more cumbersome. Three methods that can be used to estimate intensity of CRE activity include (1) metabolic equivalents or METs, (2) HR response, or (3) ratings of perceived exertion (RPE) (see table 2.2). Each approach is discussed in the following paragraphs.

One MET is the amount of oxygen the body would utilize for energy production during each minute at rest. MET values represent multiples of resting energy expenditure. When participating in an activity that is six METs, the body is using six times more oxygen than at rest. Many exercise studies have been done to determine the

Table 2.2 Estimating Activity Intensity by Three Methods

Intensity	Method		
	% maximal heart rate	RPE	METs
Very light	< 35	< 10	< 2
Light	35–54	10–11	2–4
Moderate	55–69	12–13	5–7
Vigorous	70–89	14–16	8–10
Very vigorous	≥ 90	17–19	≥10
Maximal	100	20	12

Source: U.S. Department of Health and Human Services: Physical Activity and Health: A Report of the Surgeon General. Atlanta: U.S. Department of Health and Human Services, Centers for Disease Control and Prevention, National Center for Chronic Disease Prevention and Health Promotion, 1996.

Table 2.3 Common Physical Activities for Healthy U.S. Adults by Intensity of Effort Required in MET Scores and Kilocalories per Minute

Light (< 3.0 METs or < 4 kcal · min^{-1})	Moderate (3.0–6.0 METs or 4–7 kcal · min^{-1})	Hard/vigorous (> 6.0 METS or > 7 kcal · min^{-1})
Walking, slowly (strolling) (1–2 mph)	Walking, briskly (3–4 mph)	Walking, briskly uphill or with a load
Cycling, stationary (< 50 W) or for transportation (< 10 mph)	Cycling, for pleasure (> 10 mph)	Cycling, fast or racing
Swimming, slow treading or crawl	Swimming, moderate effort	Swimming, fast treading
Conditioning exercise, light stretching	Conditioning exercise, general calisthenics	Conditioning exercise, stair ergometer or ski machine
——	Racket sports, table tennis	Racket sports, singles tennis or racquetball
Golf, power cart	Golf, pulling cart or carrying clubs	——
Bowling	——	——
Fishing, sitting	Fishing, standing/casting	Fishing, in stream
Boating, power	Canoeing, leisurely (2–4 mph)	Canoeing, rapidly (> 4 mph)
Home care, carpet sweeping	Home care, general cleaning	Moving furniture
Mowing lawn, riding mower	Mowing lawn, power mower	Mowing lawn, hand mower
Home repair, carpentry	Home repair, painting	——

From Pate, R.R. et al. (1995). Physical Activity and Public Health: A Recommendation for the Centers of Disease Control and Prevention and the American College of Sports Medicine. Journal of the American Medical Association, 273(5), 402-407, p. 404.

approximate number of METs being used during various activities. These are relative numbers that reflect an "average" person's energy expenditure in certain activities. An assumption of these studies is that the person moves in efficient patterns, which may not be the case for some persons with disabilities. While the MET values can give numbers for comparison (fewer METs for walking than for playing basketball), the charts to determine energy expenditure generally reflect energy expenditure of populations without disabilities (see table 2.3).

Perhaps the most widely used way to monitor exercise intensity is HR response. For most people, there is a direct relationship between exercise intensity and HR response to exercise. Higher intensity exercise produces higher HR response. The HR response to exercise is based on predicted maximal HR. This is typically calculated by 220 – age = HR max. This value is also based on average responses of the heart to vigorous exercise.

Once a person's maximal HR is predicted, a certain percentage of that number is used as a target figure for determining exercise intensity. For many healthy people, 60% of maximal HR is used as an initial level of intensity for a given bout of aerobic exercise. For a 15-year-old healthy student with MR, the exercise intensity may be calculated to be 220 – 15 × 60% = 123 bpm. For persons who are extremely sedentary, the intensity may be reduced to 40 or 50% initially, with progressions in in-

Table 2.4   Borg Perceived Exertion Scale

Rating of perceived exertion (RPE)	Verbal description of RPE
6	No exertion at all
7	
8	Extremely light
9	Very light
10	
11	Light
12	
13	Somewhat hard
14	
15	Hard (heavy)
16	
17	Very hard
18	
19	Extremely hard
20	Maximal exertion

Borg RPE scale © Gunnar Borg 1970, 1985, 1994, 1998

Reprinted with permission from G. Borg. (1998). *Borg's Perceived Exertion and Pain Scales*. Champaign, IL: Human Kinetics, p. 47.

tensity planned over a period of time. Extremely fit persons may start at 70% maximal HR response and work to improve the duration of the exercise bout. People are taught to monitor their HR during exercise to see if they are above or below their targeted HR response. Electronic HR monitors allow instructors or participants to monitor HR response and to vary exercise intensity based on that response. These are frequently used in long-term races, such as marathons, to help act as a guide to the racer. You should monitor prior to aerobic exercise, during exercise, and immediately following the exercise bout. The quickness with which the HR returns to normal after the completion of exercise is also an indicator of aerobic fitness.

Monitoring HR is a valuable indicator of exercise intensity and useful for exercise prescription. However, the HR response may be masked by medication or compromised neural responses (e.g., with an SCI), or it may be artificially high when a person is asked to perform a very difficult movement pattern (e.g., amputee or a person with severe CP). A teacher needs to use HR response for most people, but realize there may be complications in using this as the sole determinant of response to aerobic fitness activities.

An effective, alternative approach to monitor exercise intensity is perceived exertion. The Borg Scale (Borg, 1982) has been extensively used to give a numerical rating to perceived exercise exertion (see table 2.4). This scale has been highly correlated to other physiological responses, such as HR, aerobic capacity, and ventilatory threshold. The Borg scale is a ranking of 6 to 20, the low numbers meaning very, very light exercise and 19 to 20 being very, very hard. This may be extremely valuable in teaching people when they are exercising at the appropriate intensity, particularly if monitoring HR may give inconclusive evidence of exertion. This approach has been used with various populations with disabilities, but more evidence is needed to support its use with some populations with cognitive impairments.

In addition to manipulating the intensity, frequency, and duration of activity, instructors should also give consideration to the mode (what kind?) of activity. Rhythmic, continuous activities that use large muscle groups generally are recommended for the development of CRE. Exercise that emphasizes a specific muscle group will have a greater impact on that particular muscle group. High-impact activities (e.g., running/jogging) are not recommended for people beginning an exercise program due to the increased incidence of injury with this mode. Lower impact activities—such as swimming, cycling, or walking—likely would be more appropriate for beginners. Advances in modified equipment allow many people with disabilities the opportunity to engage in aerobic exercises. For example, there are now many types of wheelchairs that allow a variety of activities (see figure 2.2). Additional information on specific activities to develop CRE is presented in a subsequent section of this chapter.

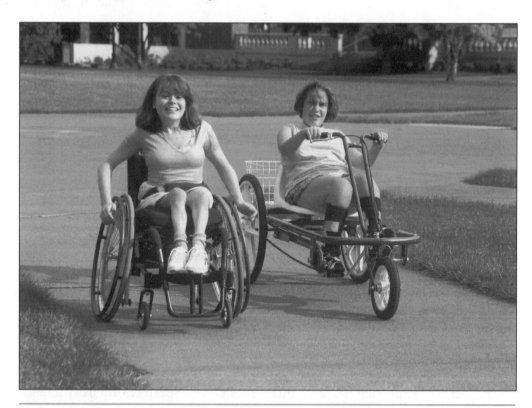

Figure 2.2 Advances in wheelchair technology enhance participation

Guidelines for the Development of Cardiorespiratory Endurance

Physical activity recommendations for the development of CRE (as well as for other components of physical fitness) have been available for many years. The ACSM, for instance, has been publishing general principles for fitness development for several years, and other recommendations can easily be found in a variety of exercise physiology texts and fitness manuals. These "exercise prescriptions" generally have been shown to be effective in improving the physical fitness of those who follow them.

More recently, however, new physical activity recommendations have emerged with a slightly different goal. These new guidelines have been called "lifetime activity recommendations" (Corbin and Pangrazzi, 1996). The cornerstone of these new recommendations is a joint statement from the Centers for Disease Control and Prevention (CDC) and the ACSM pertaining to physical activity and health (Pate et al., 1995). Contained in this paper is the recommendation that all Americans accumulate at least 30 minutes of moderate-level physical activity on most, preferably all, days of the week. The goal of such activity is not to improve CRE per se (although it may do so) but rather to directly improve the participant's health status. The paper includes scientific data documenting the relationship between physical activity and health and provides a rationale for the recommendation. Emphasis on moderate-level activity is significant because exercise prescriptions traditionally have advocated a more "vigorous" approach.

As demonstrated in figure 1.1, physical activity can contribute to both health and physical fitness. Recommendations for frequency, intensity, and duration of physical activity, however, may vary somewhat depending on the goal of the activity program. For instance, lower levels of physical activity (especially intensity) may reduce the risk of acquiring certain diseases but might not be of sufficient quality and quantity to improve $\dot{V}O_2$max (ACSM, 1998). Consequently, the reader should know that the goal of the physical activity recommendations contained in this chapter is to enhance CRE. As such, greater emphasis is placed on the guidelines associated with the more traditional exercise prescriptions. Where appropriate, however, the recommendations from the ACSM paper (and related literature) are integrated into these guidelines to acknowledge the physical activity-health connection. Emphasis was placed on the relationship between activity and fitness (i.e., exercise prescriptions) because (1) this manual was written to support physical fitness development in conjunction with the BPFT; (2) the activity recommendations for fitness generally are more rigorous than those for health, so both goals likely can be met through the fitness recommendations; and (3) health benefits can also be attained by achieving certain levels of physical fitness (critical values of $\dot{V}O_2$max or percent body fat, for instance).

The BPFT general physical activity guidelines for improving CRE among youngsters ages 10 to 17 are summarized in table 2.5. The rationale for these recommendations is discussed in the following paragraphs. In many cases these recommendations are just as appropriate for youngsters with disabilities as they are for nondisabled youngsters. Possible adjustments to the guidelines for youngsters with disabilities, however, are presented later in this section.

Adolescents

Youngsters ages 13 to 17, minimally, should engage in moderate physical activity on most, preferably all, days of the week, for at least 30 minutes per day. Ideally, at least some of the adolescent's activity should be of a more vigorous nature (Pangrazzi, Corbin, and Welk, 1996) and, if it is, the minimal frequency can be reduced to three days per week and the minimal duration can be reduced to 20 minutes per day. The BPFT recommendation for frequency, therefore, is established at 3 to 5 days per week. In fact, three days per week may be the optimal frequency for moderate to vigorous activity in the sense that the value of added improvement to $\dot{V}O_2$max is smaller beyond three days per week and virtually nonexistent beyond five days per week (ACSM, 1998). Injuries also tend to increase disproportionately

Table 2.5 Guidelines for Achieving and Maintaining Health-Related Cardiorespiratory Endurance

Group	Frequency	Intensity	Duration
Adolescents (13–17)	3–5 days/week	55–90% HR max (~115–180 beats/min) 12–16 RPE 5–10 METs	20–60 min/day (accumulated; > 10 min/bout)
Older children (10–12)	4–7 days/week	55–70% HR max* (~115–145 beats/min) 12–13 RPE* 5–7 METs*	30–60+ min/day (accumulated, intermittent)
Youngsters with disabilities (10–17)	No change for those with MR, VI, CP, SCI, or CA/A	Reduce as a function of fitness level. Adjust target HR zone (THRZ) for persons using arms-only activity and persons with SCI quadriplegia	Accumulate more intermittent activity or reduce total time if necessary

*These values represent moderate physical activity; ideally this level will be exceeded to vigorous levels at times.

MR = mental retardation, VI = visually impaired, CP = cerebral palsy, SCI = spinal cord injury, CA/A = congenital anomaly/amputation

when frequency of moderate to vigorous activity exceeds five days per week (ACSM, 1998). It is further recommended, therefore, that youngsters striving for physical activity on all days of the week (per the ACSM guideline), supplement the three- to five-day recommendation with additional days of moderate, preferably "low impact," activity or by targeting different components of fitness.

The BPFT recommendation for intensity for adolescents is moderate to vigorous. Adolescents who engage strictly in moderate-level activity meet the lifetime activity recommendations, but may fall short of the goal of improving CRE. Intensity can be monitored via HR, RPE, or estimated METs described earlier in this chapter (see table 2.2).

It's recommended that adolescents accumulate a duration of 20 to 60 minutes of moderate to vigorous activity on the appropriate number of days. The word *accumulate* suggests that the activity does not need to be continuous across the entire time frame; shorter "bouts" of activity can be added together to achieve the daily recommendation for duration. For adolescents, however, it is recommended that at least some of the activity be in continuous bouts of at least 10 minutes. If adolescents engage strictly in moderate-level activities, the minimal recommendation for duration should be increased to 30 minutes, and the minimal recommendation for frequency should be increased to four days per week.

Older Children

The recommendations discussed above for adolescents do not necessarily apply to children ages 10 to 12. The Council for Physical Education for Children (COPEC) (n.d.) emphasizes that children are different than adolescents (and certainly adults) in some significant ways that impact upon physical activity recommendations. Among those concepts cited are a relatively short attention span; a tendency toward concrete rather than abstract thought; normal activity patterns that are more intermittent than continuous; a weaker relationship between physical activity and physical fitness; and a possible perception that higher intensity activities are too difficult, perhaps contributing to withdrawal from physical activity. Consequently, COPEC (n.d.) recommends that children participate in physical activity at lesser intensities, but at greater durations and frequencies, than are recommended for adolescents in table 2.5.

The BPFT physical activity guidelines presented in table 2.5 for 10- to 12-year-olds are consistent with the COPEC (n.d.) recommendations and more closely resemble the new ACSM lifetime activity recommendations than the more traditional exercise prescription recommendations. The recommendation for frequency (four to seven days per week) reflects the notion that children should participate in physical activity on all, or most, days of the week. Indices of intensity (HR, RPE, and METs) for older children all reflect moderate levels. (While moderate activity represents an acceptable, minimal, level of intensity for 10- to 12-year-olds, ideally some of their activity will be at a more vigorous level.)

It is recommended that older children participate in age-appropriate activities for at least 30 to 60 minutes each day; in fact, COPEC (n.d.) recommended "up to several hours per day" for school-aged children (p. 8). Again, it should be emphasized that participation time (i.e., duration) can be accumulated over the course of an entire day. Another important difference between the recommendations for older children and adolescents is that intermittent activity is acceptable for children, whereas more continuous activity is recommended for adolescents.

Intermittent activity consists of periods of moderate (and, preferably, some vigorous) activity, alternating with brief periods of rest and recovery. HR, for instance, may fluctuate within and below the target HR zone for intermittent activity, but would remain in the target HR zone during continuous activity.

Adjustments for Youngsters With Disabilities

As indicated earlier, the physical activity guidelines for the development of CRE presented in table 2.5 generally are appropriate for youngsters both with and without disabilities. For instance, no adjustments to frequency are recommended here for youngsters with any of the disabilities targeted in the BPFT. (Adjustments to frequency may be appropriate when youngsters have neuromuscular diseases, arthritis, or other disabilities that may require greater periods of recovery.) Physical activity on most, preferably all, days of the week is recommended for most Americans. Still, some adjustments to intensity and duration are appropriate under certain circumstances.

First of all, intensity threshold (the minimal training intensity that will lead to improvement in $\dot{V}O_2max$) is a function of the youngster's initial level of fitness. While this is true regardless of disability, instructors may find that many of their students with disabilities may begin programs with low levels of fitness. Although the ACSM recently revised their estimates for moderate intensity downward to reflect the variability of the threshold as a function of fitness (ACSM, 1998), it may be necessary initially to allow youngsters who begin at very low levels of CRE fitness to participate in physical activities at the upper end of light intensity rather than moderate (see table 2.2). Similarly, it may be necessary to accept as appropriate shorter periods of duration and/or more intermittent activity (even for adolescents) for youngsters with initially low levels of CRE fitness. As a general guideline, instructors who work with youngsters who have very low initial levels of fitness should find an intensity at which a youngster can participate for a minimum of 10 minutes (continuous or accumulated intermittent activity) per activity session.

Instructors should recognize that if they are monitoring intensity via HR and if students are engaging in arms-only kinds of physical activity (e.g., activity done while in a wheelchair), the target heart rate zone (THRZ) will need to be adjusted downward. Instructors should subtract 10 beats per minute after determining THRZ from the values in table 2.5 (older children = 105 to 135 bpm; adolescents = 105 to 170 bpm). In cases where the student has a low cervical SCI (i.e., C6 to C8) it is recommended that the THRZ be established as follows: (1) if resting HR is below 65 beats per minute, the THRZ is 85 to 105 beats per minute; or (2) if the resting HR is at or above 65 beats per minute, the THRZ is a range that is 20 to 30 beats above the resting value.

Fernhall (1997) has reported 8 to 20% lower than expected maximal HR for people with MR, although he notes that the underlying mechanism for this finding is unknown (i.e., does MR per se cause the lower rates or do other factors such as motivation explain these findings?). Instructors who monitor the intensity of youngsters with MR by using HR, therefore, may elect to adjust THRZ values downward, especially if the youngster appears to be making a good effort but with a relatively small increase in HR. A THRZ adjustment of 10 beats per minute would approximate an 8% reduction in maximal HR for youngsters in the 10 to 17 age range.

Although estimating the MET values of various activities is a useful way to establish activity intensity, it may have questionable value for youngsters with physical disabilities. MET values are established in part on assumptions regarding mechanical efficiency. Since CP, for instance, typically results in reduced mechanical efficiency, published MET values likely will seriously underestimate the actual energy cost of many activities for many youngsters with this condition. Similarly, MET estimates probably are inaccurate for spinal cord injured youngsters who participate in physical activities in wheelchairs. It is recommended, therefore, that instructors monitor the activity intensity of youngsters with physical disabilities through either HR or RPE.

The primary possible adjustment to recommendations of duration for youngsters with disabilities is to permit more intermittent activity regardless of age. Intermittent activity for youngsters with disabilities is appropriate for any number of reasons. A few examples are as follows: (1) youngsters in wheelchairs are dependent on their arms for CRE activity, and they likely will tire before those who use their legs; (2) youngsters with MR may have shorter attention spans and may require more frequent changes in activity; and (3) youngsters with CP may tire more quickly than others in a class because they may have to work at a more vigorous level due to differences in mechanical efficiency. As much as possible, however, youngsters with disabilities still should strive to meet the minimal recommendations for total accumulated activity (duration) shown in table 2.5.

BODY COMPOSITION (BC)

BC has been defined as the relative amount of muscle, fat, bone, and other tissue that composes the body. Indices of BC generally try to identify individuals who are either excessively fat or excessively lean, or who either weigh too much for their height or weigh too little. Ideal BC scores generally lie in a "healthy fitness zone," a range of scores that is neither too high nor too low. Although more sophisticated laboratory techniques exist, determining the degree of one's leanness/fatness in field settings is usually accomplished through skinfold measurements. Subcutaneous skinfold thicknesses taken at specific sites can be entered into prediction equations to estimate percent of body fat. (The standards associated with the skinfold items in the BPFT were calculated from such equations.) The appropriateness of weight for a height can be judged from height and weight tables or, as is recommended in the BPFT, through body mass index. Body mass index (BMI) is based on a weight-to-height ratio.

Although skinfolds and BMI measures are related, they do not measure exactly the same thing. BMI considers body weight from all sources (fat, bone, muscle, etc.), whereas skinfolds focus strictly on subcutaneous fat. An excessively high skinfold evaluation, for instance, would indicate that the individual is "obese." On the other hand, an excessively high BMI score indicates that the person is "overweight." It is possible for a person to be overweight but not obese, as may be the case with an individual who has highly developed musculature. Nevertheless, both skinfolds and BMI have been linked to indices of health and provide important information about BC.

Assessment of Body Composition in the Brockport Physical Fitness Test (BPFT)

In the BPFT (Winnick and Short, 1999) BC may be assessed in one of two ways: by skinfold measurements, which reflect the amount of underlying fat tissue at specific sites on the body, or via BMI, which is calculated from height and weight data. Skinfold measurements generally are preferred when assessing BC because they more accurately predict the percentage of body mass that is due to fat than does BMI. Accurate assessment of percent body fat is important because high levels of body fat are known to contribute to health impairments.

In the BPFT, skinfold measures are taken at the triceps, subscapular, and calf locations. Usually the sum of skinfolds taken at two sites (i.e., triceps plus subscapular or triceps plus calf) serves as the criterion measure of skinfolds. In some cases, however, a single measure taken at the triceps site can be used alternatively (although the prediction of percent body fat is likely to be less accurate when using just one site).

BMI is derived from the following equation:

$$\text{body weight (kg)/height}^2 \text{ (m)} \quad \text{or} \quad 704.5 \times \text{body weight (lb)/ height}^2 \text{ (in.)}$$

BMI does not predict percentage body fat as accurately as skinfolds because body weight includes contributions from bone and muscle as well as body fat. Nevertheless, a relationship between high BMI scores and certain health impairments has been established. Consequently, BMI remains a good option for the assessment of BC, especially when administering skinfolds is not possible.

Physical Activity Guidelines for Weight Loss

Although it is apparent that there is a genetic component to some forms of obesity (Rimmer, 1994), it is also true that physical activity and diet can be used to encourage weight loss. The Surgeon General has summarized research pertaining to the effects of exercise on body weight and obesity as follows:

- Physical activity generally affects BC and weight favorably by promoting fat loss while preserving or increasing lean mass.

- The rate of weight loss is positively related, in a dose-response manner, to the frequency and duration of the physical activity session, as well as to the duration (e.g., months, years) of the physical activity program.

• Although the rate of weight loss resulting from increased physical activity without caloric restriction is relatively slow, the combination of increased physical activity and dieting appears to be more effective for long-term weight regulation than is dieting alone (U.S. Department of Health and Human Services, 1996).

Clearly a sound weight loss program will include both dietary and physical activity considerations. Although some general dietary considerations for weight loss are summarized in table 2.6, a detailed treatment of nutritional issues is beyond the scope of this book. It is recommended, however, that a structured dietary plan be formulated, with the help of a physician or dietitian as necessary, and that the plan be implemented and monitored with the assistance of parents, school personnel, the youngster, and others who have regular contact with the youngster.

Table 2.6   Some Dietary Considerations to Promote Weight Loss

Restrict caloric intake to 10 kcal/lb of body weight (example: 1,600 kcal/day for a 160-lb person).

Reduce the amount of saturated fats (daily intake of fat should not exceed 30% of total calories, and saturated fats should not exceed 10% of total calories).

Increase dietary fiber and complex carbohydrates (starches) and reduce simple carbohydrates (sugars).

Use lean meats and trim excess fat.

Reduce/eliminate cooking oils and fats in the preparation of foods (substitute canola oil or olive oil).

Broil or bake foods rather than fry.

Reduce sugar and fat in all recipes.

Seek out "fat-free" and "cholesterol-free" alternatives.

Feature fruits and vegetables at snack time.

Avoid fast food restaurants.

Source: J. Rimmer, *Fitness and rehabilitation programs for special populations,* 1994.

Some resources on physical fitness combine physical activity recommendations for CRE and BC (weight loss) (e.g., ACSM, 1998). This is a logical approach because if an individual can meet the activity guidelines associated with CRE, they will also likely meet the energy expenditure recommendations associated with weight loss. With such an approach the participant can "kill two birds with one stone." It is recommended, therefore, that participants, whenever possible and appropriate, pursue the activity guidelines presented in table 2.6 to attain both CRE and weight loss goals.

There may be circumstances, however, when the goal of the activity program focuses primarily on weight loss (with less regard for CRE). In such cases, activity programs that are characterized by greater frequency and duration and moderate intensity are effective (ACSM, 1998). Recommendations for a weight loss program are summarized in table 2.7. Of particular importance is the goal of the program, which is to attain a minimal energy expenditure of 1,000 kcal per week. Perhaps the easiest way for practitioners to estimate energy expenditure in kcal is to estimate the intensity of the activity in METs. If approximate MET values are known, kcal expended per minute can be calculated from the following equation:

$$\text{kcal/min} = \text{METs} \times 3.5 \times \text{body weight (kg)} / 200$$

For example, if Mary, a 165-pound (75-kg) youngster engages in an activity with a MET rating of 6 (e.g., playing tennis), she will expend 7.9 kcal/min. She will need to play tennis (or engage in some other activity) at that intensity for about 126 minutes in order to achieve the 1,000 kcal goal for the week (1000/7.9 = 126). If Mary plays four days per week she will need to play for about 32 minutes per day to achieve the goal (126/4 = 32). Alternatively, if she engages in activities with a MET value of 4 (e.g., playing table tennis), she will burn only 5.3 kcal/min and will need to participate for about 189 minutes to reach the goal. She could, therefore, play five days per week for about 38 minutes per day to consume 1,000 kcal/week. The values associated with frequency, intensity, and duration of the program, therefore, are interrelated and may fluctuate somewhat in pursuit of the 1,000 kcal goal.

As discussed earlier in this chapter, the use of established MET values for certain activities for youngsters with physical disabilities may not be appropriate given the mechanical efficiency assumptions that underlie the MET estimates. Instructors of youngsters with physical disabilities may wish to estimate METs from HR values or RPE, rather than from published MET tables. This could be done by consulting table 2.2 in this chapter to estimate intensity equivalents among the three methods. In that table, for instance, MET values range from 5 to 7 and percent of maximal HR values range from 55 to 69 for moderate intensity. For programming purposes we can assume that the percent HR values translate to 115 to 145 beats per minute for youngsters in the 10 to 17 age range. Consequently, corresponding MET values might be roughly estimated from HR as follows: 115 to 125 beats/min = 5 METs, 125 to 135 beats/min = 6 METs, and 135 to 145 beats/min = 7 METs. Once METs have been estimated, total energy expenditure can be approximated by using the kcal/min formula.

Selection of appropriate activities (i.e., mode) is also an important variable in weight loss programming. As with activities to enhance CRE, activities to encourage

Table 2.7 Physical Activity Guidelines for Weight Loss

Age group	Frequency	Intensity	Duration
10–17	4–7 days/week	55–70% HR max (~115–145 beats/min) 12–13 RPE 5–7 METs	30–60+ min of accumulated activity per day.
Youngsters with disabilities	No change for those with MR, VI, CP, SCI, or CA/A	Reduce as a function of fitness level; adjust THRZ for persons using arms-only activity and persons with SCI quadriplegia	Accumulate more intermittent activity; try to maintain total time (reduce intensity rather than duration as necessary)

Goal: to attain a caloric expenditure of 1,000 kcal/week (minimally).

MR = mental retardation, VI = visually impaired, CP = cerebral palsy, SCI = spinal cord injury, CA/A = congenital anomaly/amputation

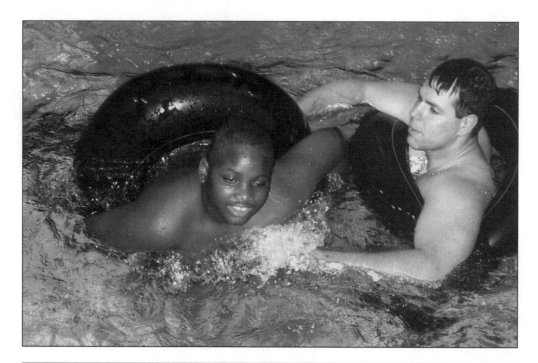

Figure 2.3 Swimming—an enjoyable activity for cardiorespiratory development and weight loss

weight loss should use large muscles, be rhythmic in nature, and allow for continuous participation. Since one of the goals of any physical activity program is to promote a physically active lifestyle, the activities selected must be enjoyable to the participant (see figure 2.3). Swimming, rowing, jogging, wheeling, dancing, cycling, hiking, cross-country skiing, and walking are just some of the activities that traditionally have been recommended for weight loss. Additional characteristics of a desirable training program for youngsters who are obese are presented in table 2.8.

Table 2.8   Characteristics of a Desirable Training Program for Youngsters Who Are Obese

Emphasizes use of large muscle groups in low-impact aerobic activities

De-emphasizes intensity, emphasizes duration

Raises daily total energy expenditure

Daily, or near-daily exercise

Gradual increase in frequency and volume

Uses well-liked activities

Recognizes that participation time can be accumulated and that intermittent activity is preferred for children

Encourages family involvement

Involves partners and/or small groups

PHYSICAL ACTIVITY CONSIDERATIONS FOR YOUNGSTERS WITH DISABILITIES

Possible adjustments to frequency, intensity, and duration of activity for youngsters with disabilities were discussed earlier in this chapter. Additional considerations related to the implementation of activities for CRE and appropriate levels of BC are presented here. They include, as appropriate, safety precautions, medical concerns, types of activities (i.e., mode), contraindications, and, in some cases, teaching methods. Finding age-appropriate activities with peers is critical. Encouraging participation in typical activities of peers will increase the likelihood of ongoing participation.

Spinal Cord Injury (SCI), Including Spina Bifida

Due to lack of sensation in the lower limbs, instructors should monitor the youngster's skin for the development of pressure sores (i.e., decubitus ulcers). Out-of-chair activities are recommended, and youngsters should be encouraged to relieve pressure on the buttocks and posterior thighs for at least five seconds every 15 minutes (e.g., perform a seated push-up). The development of blisters or skin abrasions should also be monitored.

The ability of the body to regulate heat may be impaired with SCI, thus requiring extra caution during prolonged activity or activity conducted in extreme hot/cold conditions. Appropriate clothing, adequate fluids, and attention to wind and sun exposure are important in maintaining body temperature (i.e., thermoregulation).

Active youngsters with SCI are susceptible to overuse injuries, particularly of the wrists, elbows, and shoulders. Instructors should vary the mode of activity as much as possible and encourage "cross-training." Activities that promote muscle balance and flexibility around a joint also are recommended. When some leg function exists, activities that require both arm and leg action are desirable.

Youngsters with high spinal cord lesions may need to be strapped into their wheelchairs to promote stabilization and/or may require special adaptations on the wrists or hands to assist in safe gripping of exercise equipment.

Hypotension, or low blood pressure, can occur during exercise when blood "pools" in inactive legs. This pooling can result in the early onset of fatigue and/or a feeling of light-headedness. It may be helpful to encourage youngsters to wear compression garments (hose, long socks, tights, etc.) to decrease blood pooling and to improve blood pressure.

Autonomic dysreflexia is a dangerous condition that can result in elevated blood pressure, higher HR, sweating, headache, nausea, and flushed skin for persons with lesions above T6. It can be brought on by the presence of pressure sores or by a distended bladder. Youngsters should be encouraged to empty bowel and bladder prior to participating in physical activity, and care should be taken to provide appropriate cushioning and skin pressure relief.

Some youngsters with spina bifida have latex sensitivity, likely due to long-term and early exposure to multiple forms of latex gloves. In these cases it will be necessary to avoid the use of latex-based equipment (e.g., balloons, some rubber balls, some HR monitors, etc.) in activity programs.

Cerebral Palsy (CP)

Inefficient movement due to incoordination limits physiological potential. Thus, persons with CP have higher energy expenditure to do otherwise simple tasks. This has been demonstrated with higher HR, blood pressure, and lactate concentrations for given submaximal work and slightly lower aerobic capacity (10 to 20%). Thus for many persons with CP, functional limitations for aerobic activity are due to poor movement patterns. While aerobic activity will help to increase aerobic fitness, inefficient movement will still negatively affect aerobic performance on some tasks.

Low fitness may also be a result of poor exercise habits, muscle imbalance, and poor functional strength. It is imperative for teachers to plan well-rounded exercise programs that include flexibility, aerobic capacity, and strength-related activities. Visual impairments, seizure disorders, hearing and speech impairments, and MR frequently are associated with CP. An instructor needs to recognize that these characteristics may occur, yet such educational needs *should not* be assumed for all with CP.

Due to incoordination in CP youngsters, there may be a need for strapping feet and/or hands to equipment (e.g., pedals or hand grips) for physical activity. This can be done simply with Velcro straps, or more elaborately with straps connected to equipment or to the wheelchair frame to provide greater stability. Balance may be negatively affected as one fatigues. More intense activities should occur in the earlier part of the lesson. Fatigue during activity may temporarily affect spasticity, increasing symptoms and decreasing functional ability and coordination. Youngsters should perform slow, prolonged stretching routines prior to aerobic activity.

At times, persistence of primitive reflexes may impede a person's ability to perform some activities. Proper positioning (e.g., maintaining the head in a midline, or neutral, position) and activity selection may help to minimize the effects of reflexes.

Amputations

Site and level of amputation must be considered when selecting a type of activity program for amputees. With an increase in exercise and physical activity, care should be given to check the residual stump for sores. Skin care is essential to maintain good integrity of the prosthesis. If sores persist, the person may not be able to use the prosthesis for daily activities, thereby reducing any functional benefits from exercise.

Select a type of exercise that works physically and psychologically for the person. With an upper extremity amputation, using bicycles, treadmills, stair climbers, and walking can be encouraged as forms of aerobic exercise. For a person with a lower extremity amputation, bicycling can often be adapted with a toe clip on the nonaffected side to ease the push-pull of bicycling. Most forms of walking and jogging are encouraged. However, adequate protection and frequent inspection of the skin is necessary and should be encouraged by the instructor.

Swimming is also encouraged for students with amputations. Stroke technique modifications may be needed to encourage swimming as a form of activity to improve fitness. For many with upper extremity amputations, swimming sidestroke with the more functional side down helps mobility in the water.

Focus on proper body alignment, with particular emphasis on reduction of lower back stress for persons with lower body amputations. Finding alternative ways to balance during exercise (e.g., seated) may enable the person to work at a higher workload without fear of falling.

Mental Retardation (MR)

In exercise testing, the task may be difficult to understand, and therefore the instructor may not be able to elicit true physiologic response to activity from the youngster. Many persons with MR need more supervision and instruction to learn and complete activities. Instructor effort must be directed at providing reinforcement for successful participation. Age-appropriate social reinforcements are preferred. Instructors should work as a team, including each other and parents or caregivers to identify reinforcement strategies that work for each youngster.

Since cardiac abnormalities are more common in persons with Down's syndrome, physician approval for moderate to vigorous physical activity is recommended. Few, if any, limitations should be expected. Seizures are also more common for persons with MR, so instructors should be aware of effective ways of responding should a seizure occur during or after physical activity.

Many persons with MR enjoy group participation with peers. Age-appropriate activities are preferred for this population. It is highly valued to have appropriate alternative activities and to provide choices for persons with MR. A good instructor should try to encourage the development of skills in more than one alternative for aerobic exercise. This way, as the student becomes older he or she can make choices of type/mode of activity (e.g., bicycling or swimming). Community programs need to be accessible and available. Instructors should communicate and work with community recreation leaders to facilitate after school and lifetime participation in physical activity. Efforts to get family or group home staff involved may help in motivation and adherence. Programs such as Let's Play to Grow, developed by Special Olympics International have been successful.

Motivational techniques are key, and the use of an ongoing token economy system may be necessary. Positive social praise is needed, and motivational techniques should be socially appropriate for age of participant.

Visual Impairments

Instructors should be sure to orient persons to the environment prior to activity to gain their confidence for activity setting safety. Using partners as sighted guides and coparticipants in an activity is recommended. This can facilitate social interaction, increase activity opportunities, and provide for greater feedback. Tactile cues are often sufficient to assist in successful activity participation. Running activities may require the use of a guide wire, rope, or running partner.

"Closed" activities, or those activities performed in a consistent, repeatable environment (e.g., swimming, track, bowling, and archery), are often good activities to start with for early success. Instructors should use kinesthetic teaching cues. Primary emphasis should be to identify enjoyable activities that a person with a visual impairment may do safely with friends and family. Lifetime participation is more likely when one participates with others (see figure 2.4).

Arthritis

Due to the pain often associated with juvenile forms of arthritis, the participant needs to be highly motivated, so choosing fun, reinforcing activities is recommended. There is often a chronic cycle of disuse atrophy and reduced range of motion (ROM). Activities may need to be low impact, such as swimming, aqua jogging, cross-country skiing, stationary bicycling, using an ergometer for both arms and legs, and using isokinetic resistance exercise equipment. These activities reduce stress on joints and enhance exercise within limits of pain. Encourage low-intensity exercise with shorter, more frequent bouts interspersed with rest to avoid exacerbating inflammation in the joints.

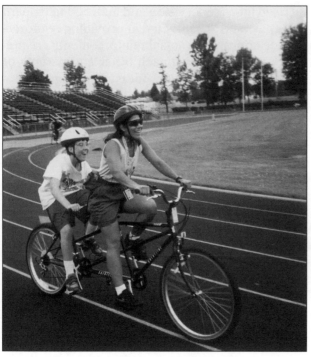 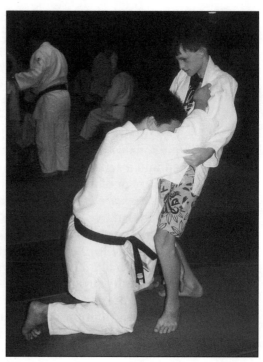

a   b

Figure 2.4a–b Good partner activities for youngsters who are blind: (*a*) tandem cycling and (*b*) judo

Prolonged warm-up and cool-down periods are critical. Instructors need to allow sufficient time to warm up prior to activities and allow time to cool down following exercise. Physician follow-up is recommended for participants with arthritis who are initiating an exercise program for the first time. Participants should recognize that some muscle-related soreness may occur, particularly when starting an exercise program. An increase in joint soreness should not last longer than one hour after an exercise bout, and if so, modification of the exercise intensity should be considered in the next exercise session (Ike, Lampman, and Castor, 1989).

Progressive Neuromuscular Disease

Muscular fatigue often occurs before the aerobic system can be trained, and thus, programs might need to focus more on the development of aerobic behavior, muscle endurance, or peak power and less on aerobic capacity.

Many forms of muscular dystrophy are progressive, and it is important to monitor the person's exercise program frequently, with formal assessment three to four times per year. This assessment should include time and distance walks or pushes to compare previous performance over similar conditions. Level of perceived exertion, as well as time to complete a given distance (e.g., a half-mile walk), would give two sources of information to monitor aerobic activity.

Contracture of the joints may be a problem if the person does not get daily exercise. Thus, flexibility-related activities are important. Physical education teachers could include flexibility exercises in class. For some, this may mean transferring out of the wheelchair to the floor for long-leg sitting and low-body stretching.

In later stages of some forms of dystrophy, respiratory muscles are affected, so diaphragmatic breathing exercises should be encouraged. Activities such as deep breathing and blowing out may be implemented. These activities can easily build into skills used while under water or for rhythmic breathing exercises.

Avoid overfatigue in these students. Build in rest periods within and between exercise sessions and evaluate levels of fatigue on days following bouts of exercise. Nutritional counseling is important since caloric expenditure is difficult in later stages of disease. Early prevention of obesity with appropriate nutrition and activity is preferred.

The effect of exercise on self-esteem is critical. Activities need to be age-appropriate and enjoyable. Teachers should be most concerned about planning activities in which the student can be interested and successful. Leisure time often becomes more sedentary as the disease progresses, but efforts to modify physical activity can help persons continue to participate in activities of daily living (ADLs). Swimming is an excellent form of exercise because the reduced effect of gravity often increases the person's potential for movement while in the water. This may allow for resistance-related training using the water as a form of resistance, as well as a potential for aerobic-type exercise in the pool.

Hearing Impairments

Community-based programs need to be made easily available to persons who are deaf. This can be done, in part, by improving communication (telephones with telecommunication devices for the deaf [TDDs] and written regulations for use of facilities).

Use alternate forms of communication including American Sign Language or gestures. Have visual cues for signaling when to start and stop the activity, shift focus for the class, or to communicate a time for questions from the students. Effective modeling is often all the communication that is needed. Instructors may be able to communicate simple commands by demonstration. However, ongoing social interaction often needs more elaborate ways to communicate. Social interaction between students needs to be prioritized during physical education.

Peers can also be effective communicators during physical education class to assist with demonstrating and interpreting a teacher's verbal instructions. Balance may be affected in some students with hearing deficits, but only when the vestibular apparatus of the inner ear is the cause of the hearing loss. Providing an opportunity for physical activity is a key factor in the development of physical fitness.

ACTIVITIES FOR CARDIORESPIRATORY ENDURANCE AND WEIGHT LOSS

Much of this manual is dedicated to the promotion of physically active lifestyles among youngsters both with and without disabilities. Physical activity can take many forms. Shephard (1994) suggests that physical activity can be categorized by occupational activity ("work"), domestic chores, required programs of physical education, and leisure activity (exercise, sport, training, dance, and play). Figure 1.1 reflects this type of categorization, although it focuses on activities conducted in physical education and leisure settings. The key point is that any activity conducted in accord with the frequency, intensity, and duration guidelines contained in this chapter will contribute to the development of CRE and BC (i.e., weight reduction) and will meet "lifetime activity recommendations." Consequently, instructors have a wide range of activity possibilities from which to choose when attempting to develop youngsters' physical fitness.

When planning programs, instructors must consider what will increase the chances that participants will continue to engage in physical activity. One of the goals of any health-related fitness program would be for youngsters to learn to incorporate physical activity into their personal lifestyles. Participating in activities that are fun is an important way of moving toward that goal. Some suggestions that teachers and other program leaders may implement to contribute to continued participation in physical activity follow.

For most children and adolescents, participation in games, sports (individual, dual, team), and other recreational pursuits that have a lifetime emphasis are especially desirable ways to make activity both enjoyable and potentially repeatable. In offering guidelines for older children (ages 10 to 12), COPEC (n.d.) indicates that participation in aerobic activities of long duration should not be emphasized. Although some youngsters may choose activities of longer duration, most will voluntarily choose participation in shorter periods of activity and instead accumulate recommended levels of physical activity. COPEC (n.d.) guidelines indicate that emphasis on conditioning for sport is premature for this group. Instead, developmentally appropriate activities are encouraged. Examples of age-appropriate developmental activities for children may include jump rope activities, relay races, obstacle courses, climbing activities (e.g., jungle gym or monkey bars), active lead-up games, active games of low organization, and rhythmic activities including creative dance and "moving to music."

Adolescents (ages 13 to 17) generally will respond more favorably than children to sport-related conditioning or training activities, however, developmentally appropriate activities with a lifetime emphasis still should be an important part of the program. Examples of activities to stimulate CRE and encourage weight loss for adolescents include fast walking, jogging or running, swimming, skiing, racket sports, basketball, soccer, skating, cycling, rowing, hiking, parcourse (i.e., fitness trail) activities, and aerobic dance or aerobic aquatics.

While many activities recommended for nondisabled youngsters also are appropriate for youngsters with disabilities, there certainly will be some differences. Instructors must consider the nature of the disability when selecting, modifying, or "inventing" activities. Some ideas for youngsters using wheelchairs might include slalom courses, freewheeling, speed bag work (i.e., rhythmically hitting an overhead punching bag), arm ergometry, seated aerobics, and active wheelchair sports (e.g., sledge hockey, basketball, track, rugby, and soccer) (see figure 2.5). When programming for youngsters with physical disabilities, instructors should select activities that require movement in both impaired and nonimpaired body parts (unless contraindicated) and activities conducted both with and without assistive devices (e.g., crutches, canes, or walkers). See table 2.9 for additional suggestions for enhancing participation. Youngsters with visual impairments might participate in activities such as calisthenics, rowing, stationary or tandem cycling, wrestling or judo, tug-of-war, step aerobics, aerobic dance, gymnastics, swimming, and track.

The ACSM (1998) has made a few important points with regard to the mode of activity. First, the ACSM points out that although a variety of activities can contribute to weight loss and the development of CRE, the effects of activity will be specific to the muscle groups used (e.g., arms and shoulders for arm ergometry, quadriceps for cycling, etc.). Consequently, the ACSM suggests that cross-training with a variety of activities may be a beneficial way of achieving a training effect. Second, the ACSM notes that both beginning and long-term participants experience more debilitating injuries as a result of high-impact activities (e.g., running, jumping) than low-impact activities (e.g., swimming, cycling), so instructors should select activities accordingly and monitor participants for musculoskeletal inju-

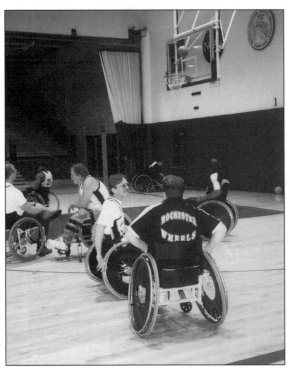 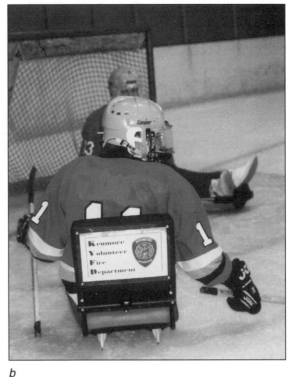

a   b

Figure 2.5a–b Aerobic activities for youngsters using wheelchairs: (*a*) basketball and (*b*) sledge hockey

ries. Finally, the ACSM observes that although resistance training alone will result in only small increases in aerobic fitness, resistance activities are recommended as part of a complete physical activity program because they have been shown to increase muscular strength and endurance and physical function. There is also speculation that resistance training conducted before initiating aerobic conditioning may reduce the possibility of injury associated with high-impact activity (ACSM, 1998).

Table 2.9   Suggestions to Enhance Participation in Physical Activity

Select well-liked activities that are developmentally appropriate.

Emphasize that accumulated physical activity is beneficial.

Give guidance regarding amount of activity, intensity, and duration.

Start easy—progress gradually.

Teach skills for lifetime activities.

Play in pleasant surroundings.

Provide for individualized and personalized attention.

Encourage self-assessment and self-monitoring.

Provide feedback regarding physiological and/or functional changes.

Develop knowledge, understanding, and values regarding health-related fitness.

Develop and implement award systems and other incentives for participation.

3

Muscular Strength and Endurance

Patrick DiRocco

When the federal government established educational rights for individuals with disabilities through the passage of federal mandates in 1975, physical education was listed as a direct service. The intent of Congress was that all children with a disability who were receiving special education services should have available to them physical education designed to meet their unique needs. Subsequent reauthorizations have maintained this intent.

The development of physical fitness is an important objective in a physical education program. An aspect of physical fitness that is related to the overall performance of the body is muscle functioning. Our muscles have the capacity to contract and extend. The extensibility of a muscle is primarily related to flexibility and to the range of motion (ROM) of our joints. This topic is discussed in chapter 4. The focus of this chapter is the force production capability of our muscles. Force production is concerned with power, strength, and muscular endurance. Strength and muscular endurance are primary concerns when developing health-related physical fitness; thus, the Brockport Physical Fitness Test (BPFT) includes measures to determine the strength and muscular endurance of youngsters. These two factors will be the primary focus of this chapter.

Since muscles move our body, sufficient strength and endurance within our muscle tissues is directly related to how effectively we will move. A severe deficit in either of these factors will reduce physiological and functional abilities. A major purpose of special education services is to help individuals to be healthy and to be as independent as possible in their activities of daily living (ADLs). Thus, for physical educators or others working with persons who have a disability, it is important to provide a systematic program that will help maintain and, when possible, improve muscular strength and endurance.

This chapter presents information on how a professional can help individuals with disabilities to better produce force and to sustain repetitive force exertion. Following an introduction, basic concepts of muscle action and muscle physiology are presented. Next is a section identifying factors impacting on training and suggestions for achieving a positive training effect. General and specific considerations for developing and maintaining muscular strength and endurance for individuals with selected disabilities is a major section in the chapter. Finally, guidelines for developing and maintaining health-related physical fitness are discussed and recommended.

Before beginning, it should be remembered that strength and muscular endurance is one aspect of a person's physical fitness and that this component does not work in isolation. Strength and muscular endurance constantly interact with flexibility, aerobic functioning, motor skill, and nutrition to produce a functional skill. A person's physical fitness development should not exclusively involve the development of strength and muscular endurance.

BASIC CONCEPTS OF MUSCLE ACTION

All muscles are attached to bones. The attachment on the body segment that will anchor the muscle is known as the origin, whereas the attachment on the body segment that will be moved by the muscle is called the insertion. The line of pull of the muscle is between the origin and insertion and creates the body segment movement that is observed. The primary movements created by muscles are flexion, in which the joint angle between two body parts is decreased; extension, in which the joint angle between two body segments is increased; adduction, which occurs when a body part is moved toward the center of mass; abduction, which occurs when a body part is moved away from the center of mass; internal rotation, in which a limb is rotated medially; and external rotation, in which a limb is rotated laterally.

Muscle action occurs through the contraction of muscle fibers. There are two types of contractile actions. When contraction of a muscle results in the shortening of the length of that muscle, that action is known as a concentric contraction. This will occur when a muscle is involved as a prime mover. Thus, the muscles of the upper arm that create elbow flexion are creating this action through concentric contractions. When there is contraction in a muscle during the lengthening of that muscle, the contractile action is known as eccentric contraction. This action occurs when there is a need to control the speed at which a joint is moved. Thus, when lowering a cup of coffee to a table by extending the forearm, the biceps, through eccentric contraction will be helping to control the speed of the action.

There are three aspects that resistance training attempts to improve. The first is the element of strength. Strength refers to the maximum capability of a muscle to generate force. This is measured by observing the maximum force production in a single movement. For example, the maximum amount of weight a person can move while doing a forearm curl would represent the strength of the muscle group that produces that action. The second element of force production is muscular endurance. Muscular endurance refers to the capacity of a muscle to produce repetitious actions at a given submaximal strength level. This is assessed by observing the maximum number of repetitions that can be produced at a submaximal intensity level. For example, the maximum number of sit-ups that a person can do before needing to stop and rest would represent the muscular endurance of the muscle group that produces the action. The third element affected by training is that of power. Power refers to the speed needed to produce a muscular contraction. Thus, whenever a forceful movement is required to occur quickly, the element of power is involved. For example, rising from a chair or popping a wheelchair over a curb would be a power action (Lockette and Keyes, 1994).

During movement, muscles conduct various functions to enhance movement efficiency (Lockette, 1995). This needs to be kept in mind when assessing the functional capacity of persons with a disability so that the best training program can be determined. The muscles that produce the primary force for a movement are known as the prime movers (agonists). The muscles that produce the opposite action are known as antagonists, and they are inhibited from contracting to allow the prime action to occur. However, as was explained above for eccentric contractions, these muscles are sometimes used to control the speed of an action. Muscles can also be assistors when the movement is against heavy resistance. These muscles do not provide the main force for the action, but are used when the work is highly intensive. A muscle can also act as a stabilizer during a movement. These muscles stabilize other bones and joints to allow an action to occur. An example is kicking. The plant foot needs to be stabilized so that the kicking leg can be swung forward. The fifth function a muscle can engage in during a movement is as a synergist. This occurs when muscles are involved in creating more than one movement. For example, the hamstrings produce both knee flexion and hip extension. When knee extension is desired without hip flexion, the hamstrings, which do not produce knee extension, will contract to reduce hip flexion.

BASIC MUSCLE PHYSIOLOGY

Training effects occur through changes that are obtained based on muscle physiology. This section is designed to present information on how muscles react to training so that training techniques are best understood. This section includes information dealing with basic structure and control mechanisms, effects of training, and anaerobic metabolism.

Basic Structure and Control Mechanisms

Muscle tissue is composed of bundles of individual fibers. There are three basic fiber types (see table 3.1). The first type is known as slow twitch (ST) because they are fatigue-resistant fibers. These fibers support long-duration exercise activity. ST fibers are also referred to as Type I fibers. These fibers have a slow speed of contraction, a low rate of fatigue, and a low strength of contraction. The second type of fibers is known as fast twitch (FT), and they primarily support muscle activity that requires strength and power. FT fibers have a fast speed of contraction, a high rate of fatigue, and a high strength of contraction. These fibers are also referred to as Type IIb fibers. The third type of fiber, known as Type IIa, is called an intermediate fiber. This fiber type is a subgroup of the FT fibers. They have a fast speed of contraction, an intermediate rate of fatigue, and a high strength of contraction. The distribution of fiber types is genetically determined; however, based upon the function of a muscle, one type will dominate (Fleck and Kraemer, 1997).

Muscles are innervated by the peripheral nervous system. A motor unit is a group of fibers that are innervated by a single motor neuron. All the fibers in a

Table 3.1   Description of Basic Muscle Fiber Types

Type	Contraction speed	Fatigue rate	Contraction strength
Slow twitch: Type I	Slow	Low	Low
Intermediate: Type IIa	Fast	Intermediate	High
Fast Twitch: Type IIb	Fast	High	High

motor unit are the same type. Generally speaking, muscles used for more fine motor movements have a higher percentage of ST fibers, and muscles used mostly in gross motor movements will be composed of more FT fibers.

When muscle fibers contract, they are only capable of contracting maximally. When a motor unit is innervated, all the fibers in that unit will contract simultaneously and with maximum force. This is known as the all-or-none principle. The more force that an action requires, the more motor units that are recruited to complete the task (Fleck and Kraemer, 1997).

Effects of Training

The initial increase in strength that is observed in trained muscles is most likely due to neural adaptations. The neural adaptations are probably a combination of increased motor neuron excitability, increased activation of synergists, and an increased inhibition of the antagonist muscles (Fleck and Kraemer, 1988). After six to eight weeks of systematic training, fiber adaptations will occur. These adaptations will have a positive effect upon the force production capabilities of the muscle groups that are being trained. Although there is agreement that muscles increase in size as a result of strength training, there are differences of opinion on how the muscles increase in size. One view is that the cross-sectional area of muscle fibers increases, and the other attributes enlargement to an increase in the number of muscle fibers. Most physiologists believe that the increase in muscle size is due to the enlargement of muscle fibers (Howley and Franks, 1997).

While an increase in strength will be a positive effect of training, one immediate effect of training that the teacher will need to understand is postworkout soreness (Lockette and Keyes, 1994). This is a by-product of the muscle engaging in an overexertion state during the workout. This overexertion probably produces some trauma at the muscle fiber and connective tissue level that will need to be repaired. Highly intensive exercise/activity sessions may produce soreness immediately following the workout. Unless there are circulation problems present, the soreness will usually decrease within one to two hours. More frequently, individuals will experience delayed soreness. This soreness will occur 24 to 48 hours following the workout. How long the soreness lasts depends on the extent of the overexertion. Once people get into a regular exercise/activity routine, the presence of delayed soreness usually goes away. For individuals who engage in regular exercise/activity, delayed soreness is present only when a muscle group is greatly overexerted (Miller, 1995). It is important that the teacher understands the possible existence of postexercise soreness and does two things. First, for new participants, the planned workout is of a moderate intensity, so that the delayed soreness is not so severe that the next workout is impaired. Secondly, the teacher should inform the person that soreness may occur and why it is present to avoid the possibility that the person would be intimidated from performing future workouts.

Anaerobic Metabolism

Muscles need to use energy in order to do work. The body uses chemical energy in the form of adenosine triphosphate (ATP) to generate the energy it needs. ATP can be reformed and used with or without the presence of oxygen. The chemical processes used when oxygen is not present is known as anaerobic metabolism. This type of metabolism is used when the exercise/activity is of a short duration and in many cases high intensity, such as resistance training or sprinting (Fleck and Kraemer, 1997).

Anaerobic metabolism uses two energy sources. The first is the breakdown of the ATP-PC molecules to produce ATP. This source is depleted within 10 seconds. If the exercise will continue beyond that time frame, the body will use glucose to produce ATP through the process of glycolysis. Glycolysis is a precursor to aerobic metabolism, which is what the body will need to use if the exercise continues beyond two to three minutes.

Anaerobic metabolism will produce a quicker fatigue rate than aerobic metabolism due to two factors. The first is related to the percent of maximal contraction that the muscles produce. Occlusion of blood flow starts to occur around 20% of maximal contractions, and complete occlusion will occur at approximately 70% of maximal effort. Thus, if the effort is above 50%, the rate that waste products are removed is slowed and fatigue occurs faster (Miller, 1995). Secondly, glycolysis produces lactic acid as a by-product, and this substrate increases the rate of fatigue. High-intensity exercise activity will also increase the heart rate (HR), breathing rate, and blood pressure. Anaerobic metabolism produces higher heart rates per percent of oxygen uptake. These issues will be discussed later in the chapter when adjustments to particular disabilities are addressed.

Whenever repetition of action occurs, muscular endurance is present. If muscular endurance is impaired, then the capacity of a person to continue to produce the desired muscular force, over time, will be limited. However, like other aspects of force production, muscular endurance can be improved with systematic training. Metabolically, muscular endurance uses both anaerobic and aerobic systems. The muscle cells' ability to continue to generate energy, usually through glycolysis, will determine the endurance capacity of that muscle. Training methods for muscular endurance will be discussed in later sections of this chapter.

Measurement of Strength and Endurance on the Brockport Physical Fitness Test (BPFT)

A total of 16 test items are included on the BPFT to measure strength and endurance. The test items and regions of the body represented by measurements are presented in table 3.2. Although 16 possible test items are included in the test, youngsters typically are administered only two or three test items. Test item selection guides associated with various appropriate classifications or subclassifications of youngsters with disabilities present test items to be used with youngsters. Once test items are administered to individuals for whom they are

Table 3.2   Test Items Related to Muscular Strength and Endurance on the Brockport Physical Fitness Test

Test item	Regions of the body
Curl-up and modified curl-up	Abdomen
Pull-up	Upper body (particularly elbow flexors)
Modified pull-up	Upper body (particularly elbow flexors)
Flexed arm hang	Hand, arm, shoulder
Extended arm hang	Hand, arm, shoulder
Push-up	Upper body (particularly elbow extensors)
Isometric push-up	Upper body
Bench press and dumbbell press	Upper body (particularly elbow extensors)
Dominant grip strength	Hand and forearm
Trunk lift	Back
Reverse curl	Hand, wrist, arm
Seated push-up	Upper body (particularly elbow extensors)
40-m push/walk	Upper body/lower body
Wheelchair ramp test	Upper body

recommended, health-related physical fitness is evaluated on the bases of general and specific standards.

A general standard is one that is associated with the general population. It is a test score that is related to either functional or physiological health and is attainable by youngsters whose performance is not significantly limited by impairment. A specific standard also reflects functional or physiological health, but it has been adjusted in some way to account for the effects of a specific impairment on performance. General standards may be recommended for the general population and youngsters with specific disabilities. Specific standards are only provided for selected test items for specific target populations. General standards may be designated as minimal or preferred.

For bench press, dumbbell press, extended arm hang, flexed arm hang, grip strength, push-ups, pull-ups, and curl-ups, minimal general standards are used. The standards are associated with criteria established by a panel of experts or with the ability to score at or above the 20th percentile for the general population. Preferred general standards are associated with criteria extablished by a panel of experts or with the ability to score at or above the 60th percentile. For the trunk lift only, a single general standard based on expert opinion and representing a good level of fitness is used. Specific standards are used to evaluate the fitness of individuals with disabilities on the reverse curl, seated push-up, 40-meter push/walk, and the wheelchair ramp test. The bases for these standards come from their relationship to ADLs. Finally, specific standards are used to evaluate the health-related physical fitness of youngsters with mental retardation (MR) and mild limitations in physical fitness. These have been developed on the basis of performance discrepancies between youngsters who are retarded and their nondisabled peers and lead to the attainment of minimal general standards.

VARIABLES INFLUENCING THE DEVELOPMENT OF STRENGTH AND ENDURANCE

The best way to improve the body's capacity to produce force is to use a progressive training regimen. Based upon the individual's fitness level, movement capabilities, and goals, the variables within a program can be adjusted. The purpose of this section is to identify and discuss important variables associated with the development of strength and endurance in order to produce a training effect.

Overload

Once a muscle group has attained a certain strength level, it will only improve if it is overloaded, that is, worked at a greater level than its normal load. As long as the training level is not beyond the muscle's capacity to perform, continuous overload will produce physiological adjustments that will create an increase in strength and/or muscular endurance. The variables of overload include frequency, intensity, duration, and mode of exercise/activity. For strength and muscular endurance exercise training, intensity is influenced by the amount of resistance moved, the number of repetitions per set, and the rest period provided between sets, while duration is concerned with the number of sets performed. The combination of the two (intensity and duration) determines training volume. Thus, if a person is working the biceps muscle and does eight repetitions of 30 pounds and does three sets, then the total volume for the biceps muscle would be 720 pounds. Programs related to the development of strength and endurance frequently design intensity as a percentage of maximum effort. Maximum effort is considered to be the maximum amount of weight that a person could move, one time, through an exercise motion. For example, if a person's maximum load for a bench press were 150 pounds, then 70% of max would be 105 pounds. The actual effort used in an exercise is primarily based on the abilities of the individual and the objectives and goals of a program. Mode refers to the type of activity that is undertaken, including types of contraction, types of resistance, the way activities are performed, and the nature of the activity.

Concepts relating to overload can be applied to general activity programs as well as to more structured or formal exercise routines. Specific recommendations regarding frequency, intensity, duration, and mode are presented subsequently, particularly in the section on guidelines for the development of muscular strength and endurance. The intensity/duration ratio that is developed for each person is also based on established training objectives and goals. These, of course, may be influenced by limitations imposed by a disability. In subsequent sections of this chapter, specific disability-related considerations will be discussed.

Fatigue

Training may produce fatigue and soreness. The muscle needs a period of time to recover from an exercise/activity workout so that it can produce the same amount of work. A general rule is to allow a muscle a minimum of approximately 48 hours to recover. The muscle needs time to replenish its energy stores, repair fiber damage, and remove waste products that were produced by energy metabolism in order to do an equal amount of work in the next training/activity session (Fleck and Kraemer, 1997).

Range of Motion

Muscles develop strength and endurance at the angles that they are trained. In order for a muscle to increase its force production throughout the entire ROM that it acts upon, the movement of the training exercise/activity must be completed throughout the full ROM. If the motion of the exercise is less than the full ROM, then the increased force production will only occur at the shortened range. In order to exert force throughout the ROM, it is important that the resistance the individual is asked to move is manageable throughout the full ROM (Fleck and Kraemer, 1997).

Isolation

In order to maximize the effects of an exercise upon a muscle, it is important to allow the targeted muscle to do as much work as possible. For every movement of a body part, a group of muscles cooperate to achieve that action. Each individual muscle has a certain line of pull between its origin and insertion. In order to maximize the effect upon a given muscle, a specific line of pull must be emphasized during an exercise. This is referred to as isolating a muscle. In reality, the muscle does not work alone, but it works at its best angle. An example is a lateral abduction movement used to work the deltoid muscle. If the elbow is not flexed during the exercise, the deltoid is doing most of the work to lift the resistance to shoulder height. However, if the elbow is allowed to flex, then the biceps is doing some of the work to lift the resistance, and the deltoids are working less. Thus, it is important to understand the proper line of pull for a given exercise to be performed correctly during each repetition (Lockette and Keyes, 1994).

Breathing

Many individuals have a tendency to hold their breath during resistive work. This increases internal thoracic pressure and is contraindicated when performing the exercise. Exercise leaders should encourage participants to maintain rhythmic breathing during exercise. The easiest way to do this is to exhale during the hard part of the exercise and to inhale during the recovery part of the movement (Fleck and Kraemer, 1997). This is usually not a problem during participation in general physical activity sessions. Students do not usually hold their breath when engaging in games, sports, dance, or other motor activities.

Types of Contraction

The way muscles contract to perform an exercise has been an important area of study by movement scientists. Three types of contractions that have been shown to produce positive effects include isotonic, isometric, and isokinetic.

Isotonic contractions involve observable movement during which the resistance to movement is constant and the tension exerted by muscle(s) is variable. Isotonic contractions may be concentric or eccentric. An individual performing a 20-

pound arm curl exercise is engaging in an isotonic exercise. The actual tension within the muscle changes during the range of movement during the exercise. However, from a practical standpoint, the person is providing the necessary tension needed to move a certain resistance a prescribed distance. This method of exercise will provide a training effect throughout the full ROM of the joint (Fleck and Kraemer, 1997).

Isometric contractions occur when tension is developed without joint movement. This occurs when there is a pushing or pulling action against an immovable force. Thus, when persons push against a wall or push their hands together with no resultant movement, they are performing an isometric exercise. This type of exercise will produce a training effect only at the joint angles at which the exercise is performed. If a training effect is desired throughout the full ROM, then a series of isometric contractions should be performed at various angles throughout the ROM. This type of exercise should be used if joint movement is restricted due to pain or a healing period, or if lack of movement is a limitation for the individual and improved strength at a certain angle is desired. An example would be the ability to hold one's buttock one to two inches above the seat for a 5- to 10-second time period to help reduce the occurrence of pressure sores.

The third type of contraction is called isokinetic and requires specialized machines to stimulate the contraction. In isokinetic movements, resistance varies and the muscle contracts at its capacity or a constant percentage of capacity. Movements are made at a constant speed throughout the full ROM. Specialized machines, such as a Cybex, adjust the resistance throughout the range of movement so that the speed will stay constant. Like isotonic, isokinetic exercise will produce a training effect through the full ROM. If a person has the machines available, this would be an effective way to exercise; however, most teachers will not have the equipment available.

Types of Resistance

The development and maintenance of strength and endurance is influenced by types of resistance. Most teachers have had experience with the use of weights to provide resistance for muscles. Various companies manufacture machines that allow individuals to exercise against the resistance of weights. The benefits of these machines are that (1) they are safe and no spotting of the weights is needed, (2) they produce incremental resistance so individuals of various fitness levels can utilize each machine, and (3) they are set up to do a particular exercise so the instructor knows how the person will be moving.

Weight machines can also be beneficial for persons with a disability (see figure 3.1). However, due to their individual limitations, for some individuals who have a disability, weight machines are not always the best choice. Weight machines can sometimes be difficult for persons to transfer into from their wheelchairs. Machines are associated with particular movements that may be impossible for some persons with a disability to perform. The minimum weight and/or weight increments are sometimes too large for some persons with a disability. In addition, some disabilities create smaller limb lengths and/or trunk sizes for a given height. This may produce an unsafe situation, since the person's body proportions do not safely fit the machine. This is also exemplified when preadolescents attempt to use machines designed for adult proportions (National Strength and Conditioning Association [NSCA], 1996). Because of these factors, it is important to have free weights (dumbbells and barbells) available for use. Free weights also allow persons to work on their stabilizing muscles, and hand weights permit a person

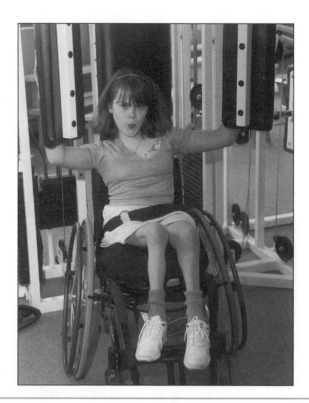

Figure 3.1 Weight machines provide convenient forms of resistance

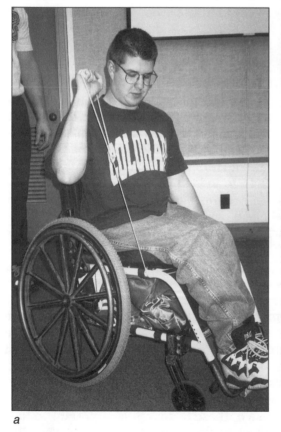

a

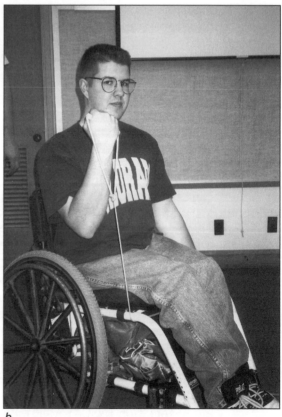

b

Figure 3.2a–b Using surgical tubing as an exercise mode: (*a*) pronated grip and (*b*) supinated grip

to work one side of the body at a given time. It is important that free weights be available so a program can be individualized.

Along with machines and free weights, teachers should have various types of tubing available for use. One type of tubing that can be used is surgical tubing, shown in figure 3.2. This type of tubing can be purchased through medical supply stores and is usually inexpensive. Tubes can provide increased resistance by increasing their diameter. Another type of tubing is thera-band and is used frequently by physical therapists. These are wide stretchable bands that can be used with many body parts in many different exercises. They provide flexibility in the process of individualizing. Bands can also be tied to hands and wrists when grips are impaired. Tubes and bands give great flexibility in designing an exercise, since they can be attached to objects, held by partners, or held by the exerciser. They permit the exercise leader freedom to create the best line of pull for each individual.

When using tubes and bands, the person should maintain an even speed throughout the exercise. This will allow individuals to effectively work their muscles in both directions. If an even speed is not maintained, the tubes or bands may snap back during the recovery part of the exercise and the person will get less work.

In addition to bands and free weights, manual resistance may be used as a resistance mode. For example, a teacher's own body parts would be used as a form of resistance (see figure 3.3 for examples of various approaches). This can be an effective exercise format that may be used with persons who are severely impaired. When using this approach the teacher would still determine the best line of pull for the muscle(s) to be worked. The teacher should provide sufficient resistance to allow the targeted muscles to work, but not to the extent that the student cannot move the body part through the functional ROM. If the student is stronger than the teacher, the student should tense the targeted muscles and, while keeping the muscles tense, move the body part through the ROM 15 to 20 times before the teacher provides resistance. This should sufficiently tire the student so that the teacher can provide adequate resistance.

Exercise Order

The order in which exercise is performed influences fatigue of a muscle group, which impacts upon the amount of work a person performs in an exercise session. The order that is selected is based on the goals of the program.

For health-related physical fitness, multijoint exercises (e.g., bench press and one-arm rows) should be done first followed by single-joint exercises (e.g., biceps curls and leg extension). This order is recommended to avoid limitation of repetitions by the larger muscle groups due to fatigue in the smaller muscles. Upper- and lower-body exercises could be alternated to allow each part of the body to recover for the next set. If the person does not have function in the lower extremities, then agonist and antagonist muscle groups could be alternated. The exercise order should be planned by the teacher so that each workout session can have maximum effect (Lockette, 1995).

If a group exercise program is being conducted, such as in a physical education class, the same concepts can be used. If materials like tubing are used and all students have their own tubing, they could do the same exercises in the same order. In this situation, it would probably be best to use partners and alternate sets. If a weight room venue is being used, it would probably be best to group students and assign each group to an exercise station. Again, group members could alternate sets before moving to the next station.

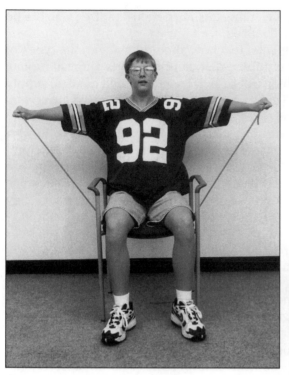

a

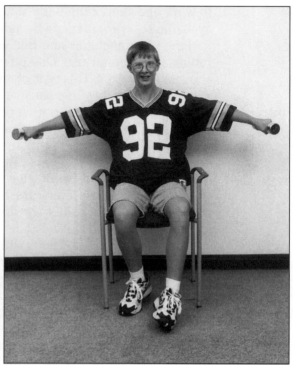

b

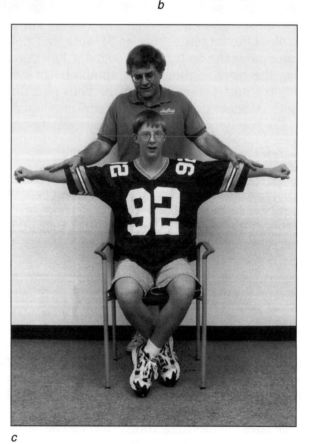

c

Figure 3.3a–c Examples of how to provide resistance (*a*) using bands, (*b*) free weights, and (*c*) manual resistance

Training Systems

Systems of training have been developed to effectively and efficiently enhance the development and maintenance of strength and endurance. They are essentially progressions and arrangements of exercise sessions in which factors affecting overload are manipulated. Although typically used by serious competitors, they can be modified for persons interested in developing health-related physical fitness through structured exercising. In this section, four systems are recommended to develop health-related fitness: basic, pyramiding, superset, and cycling. After specific exercises to be performed and the order of performance are determined, one of these systems should help achieve the goals of each individual.

1. Basic system: The person performs two to three sets of each exercise, using the same number of repetitions and load for each set. There is a three- to four-minute rest between sets.

2. Pyramiding: In this system, the person performs sets at progressively higher or lower intensities of exercise. For example, the three sets may be performed at 70, 60, and 50% maximum. A pyramid system may be a preference for a change of pace after the participant has been exercising for a few months.

3. Superset: In this system, the participant performs one set of each exercise. For example, a load of 60% could be set and the number of repetitions would be the maximum amount that could be performed at that load. In most cases, the number would be between 8 and 12. This system is desirable when time is limited.

4. Cycling: In this method, one set of each exercise would be performed with only a 15- to 30-second rest between sets. After a 5- to 10-minute rest period, a second cycle would be performed. If some cardiorespiratory benefits are also desired during the workout, this method might be preferred.

ASSESSMENT FOR INDIVIDUALIZED TRAINING

Training for the development of strength and endurance may be accomplished in individualized programs designed for that purpose. An initial assessment of the individual is important in this regard to enhance programming.

An important early step for individualized training is to determine appropriate intensity for strength development. Appropriate intensity level for each exercise in a training program is based upon one's maximum effort for each exercise. Percent of maximum effort is used to determine training volume in an exercise session. Maximum effort is defined as the maximum amount of weight that a person can move through the total distance of an exercise (ROM) only one time. It is recommended that it be estimated, since to do otherwise would be very time consuming. It would involve starting arbitrarily at a certain resistance level and then, through trial and error, determining one-repetition maximum. In addition, the trial-and-error process could put the participant at risk for an injury if the amount of weight the person attempted to lift was too heavy.

A quick and safe way to establish initial training intensity based on one-repetition maximum (one's best effort) or a percentage of one-repetition maximum is to predict it. Table 3.3 applies a prediction method that has been used in Fitness Is for Everyone clinics conducted by Disabled Sports USA. The first step in applying the prediction table is to choose a weight that the participant should be able to lift submaximally for no more than 12 repetitions and have the person lift the weight as many times as possible.

Once the repetitions are known, the prediction chart presented in table 3.3 is used to determine the percentage that corresponds with the number of repetitions completed. The weight lifted is divided by the percentage in the table to determine predicted one-repetition maximum. The predicted one-repetition maximum can then be used as a reference when setting the appropriate weight at a given level of intensity. Applying table 3.3 to an example in which the original effort resulted in lifting a 280-pound weight for five repetitions, the percentage of .857 is used to divide into 280 pounds The result is 325 and represents predicted one-repetition maximum. An individual exercising at 70% of this weight would use a weight consisting of approximately 228 pounds. While this method may not be 100% accurate, it will give a reasonably close estimate so that submaximal intensity levels used for training can be established safely and efficiently.

When working with populations with a disability, it is also important to learn in the assessment process for intensity what might be creating weakness if it exists. This information will be an important aspect in deciding what elements of strength and endurance to emphasize, which muscles to develop, and how a workout should be conducted. For example, if the weakness is due to reduced nervous system innervation of the muscle (e.g., spinal cord injury [SCI]), the impaired muscles cannot be greatly improved, and the emphasis should be on unimpaired muscle(s) that must compensate. On the other hand, if weakness is associated with a progressive muscle disorder (e.g., muscular dystrophy), the emphasis should be on maintaining current strength and the improvement of muscular endurance.

Another factor to assess is the individual's postural stability in the upright, sitting, and lying positions. This information is important for determining appropri-

Table 3.3   Repetitions and Percentages for Predicting One-Repetition Maximum

# repetitions	%
1	1.000
2	.955
3	.917
4	.885
5	.857
6	.832
7	.809
8	.788
9	.769
10	.752
11	.736
12	.721

Sample: maximum of 5 reps. with 280 lbs: 280/.857 = 325 predicted maximum.

Source: Unpublished system for determining one-repetition maximum used in Fitness is for Everyone clinics conducted by Disabled Sports USA.

ate body positioning and stabilization needs for exercise. If a person is very unstable in a position and support cannot effectively be given (e.g., strapping or support to a body part), this clearly is not a position in which a person could do quality work. Knowing stabilization needs would help in determining if it would be best to work sides of the body together rather than independently.

Observing the ROM of the joints to be involved in a program would also assist in the initial design of the program. Knowing the ROM of each joint to be moved would help in determining the best line of pull for each exercise. Also, if ROM between body sides is asymmetric, it may be more appropriate to work each side independently.

Another element to assess for individualized training is the motor control a person has of the muscles that will be exercised. An example occurs in the case of movement patterns that emerge from cerebral palsy (CP) or head injuries. Poor motor control could reduce the postural stabilization that a person has at rest, require that the exercise be performed in a different position, or require that equilibrium support assistance be given during the exercises. Some individuals with poor motor control will have difficulty performing at fast speeds and will require that all exercises be performed slowly. Inefficient control will also increase the energy cost of the movement and bring about quicker fatigue. In some cases, individuals would have to work each side of the body separately. This will be discussed in subsequent sections of the chapter.

The cause for weakness may be acquired from medical records and/or medical consultation. Postural stability can be observed by having the individual independently stand, sit, and lie in the prone and supine positions while moving arms and legs. Joint ROMs can be observed by having the person move each joint, without resistance, through its functional ROM. Motor control can be observed by having the individual do both unilateral and bilateral movements of selected parts of the body. Some of the information will be readily apparent at the initial

Table 3.4   Assessment Items for Individualized Training

Item	How/where	Why
Maximum resistance for each exercise	Estimate one-repetition maximum using a predictive process	To be able to set adequate initial intensity
Causes of weakness	Acquire information from medical records and medical consultation	To be able to set proper goals
Postural stability	Determine if a person can maintain, without help, a standing and/or sitting position	To determine if adjustments are needed
ROM of joints	Observe ROM by having person move each joint without resistance through its full ROM	To be able to recommend proper patterns for each exercise
Motor control	Observe participants' gripping ability and coordination during movement pattern(s) to be used	To be able to design proper patterns and speed to be used with each exercise

meeting with the person. For example, if the person arrives in a wheelchair and is paralyzed from the waist down, observing the balance ability and movement ability of the lower limbs is not necessary. Several pieces of information will also be gained during the performance of tasks. For example, when a person is asked to do an exercise for the purpose of determining one-repetition maximum, that person's postural stability, ROM, and motor control of the muscles and joints involved in the movement will also be observed. Although preliminary assessment must consider the areas discussed earlier, initial assessment does not have to involve an independent test for all the elements discussed above. See table 3.4 for a listing of information that should be gathered and examples of how each piece of information could be independently acquired.

A GENERAL ACTIVITY APPROACH

Although muscular strength and endurance can be developed and maintained in a formal exercise program, it can also be enhanced by engaging in general physical activities (active play, games, sports, ADLs, etc.). In fact, age and developmen-

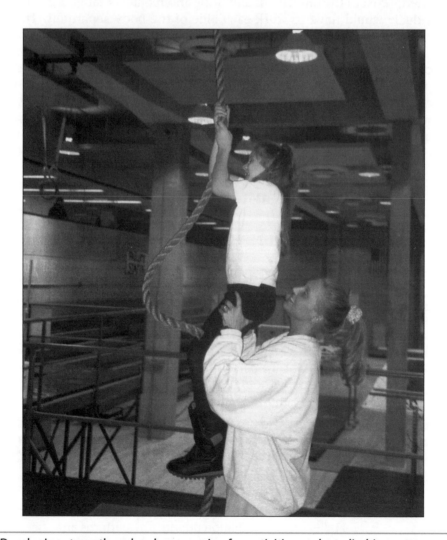

Figure 3.4 Developing strength and endurance using fun activities, such as climbing a rope

tally appropriate activities (see figure 3.4) rather than formal exercises and conditioning programs may be most important for the development of health-related physical fitness for children and adolescents, since they typically are more fun to perform and sustain. To produce a training effect over time, however, the activities would have to create an overload for the muscles. Examples of activities for younger children include developmental playground activities (horizontal ladder, chinning bar, jungle gym, etc.); combatives (tug-of-war, hand and leg wrestling); stunts; self-testing activities (rope climb, long jumping); animal walks; tumbling activities; swimming and other aquatic activities; and individual, partner, and group games involving force exertion. For adolescents, many of these activities, as well as increased involvement in higher-level sports and recreational activities, can be pursued. Rock climbing, cycling, canoeing, rowing, skiing, hunting, football, archery, wrestling, weight lifting, and track and field events are but a few of the activities and sports involving strength and endurance.

Muscle groups of the shoulder, arms, abdomen, and legs are among those that can be developed in general activity settings. Table 3.5 includes examples of activities that can be used to develop the strength and muscular endurance of these areas of the body. In a physical education class setting, strength and muscular endurance activities typically are included as a portion of the class. In this setting, relay races, station work, individual activities, circuits, and obstacle courses may be included as activities. Table 3.6 presents an example of individualized station work for the development of strength and endurance. Creative and novel tasks will motivate students to work harder. Accumulation of daily or weekly points toward a long-term goal frequently enhances motivation.

Table 3.5 Classroom Activities for Developing Strength and Endurance

Body area	Movements	Activities
Shoulders	Lift object overhead	Hold medicine ball with two hands and lift the arms from chest level to an overhead position with straight arms.
Arms	Push	Push a medicine ball across a table to a partner.
	Pull	Lying supine at the end of a matted surface that is extended 15 feet from stall bars, pull the body across the mat by pulling along a rope that is attached to the stall bars.
	Climb	Climb stall bars to designated spot without using legs.
Abdomen	Raise trunk forward	In a supine position, knees bent, bell extended over knees, raise upper trunk off the floor until bell can be rung with the hands.
Legs	Push	Sitting next to a large weighted box, push a box across a designated distance with the legs.
	Pull	Pull a weight box with a rope a designated distance.
	Climb	On a matted area, climb stacked bolsters to the top and down the other side.

Table 3.6   A Sample of Individualized Station Work for the Development of Strength and Endurance

Organization
Separate the class into three groups. Have each group start at a different station and move to the next station at the teacher's signal. While at a station, each student will perform tasks individually. Each student will have an individual card stating their task and a place to record their performance.

Station 1

At this station, the students will do tasks 1 and 2. Equipment at this station will include various sized hand weights, tubing, and weighted plastic jugs. Students choose equipment for their particular exercises.

Task 1   Work on shoulder muscles by grasping a weight with two hands at waist level. Keeping arms straight, raise weight above head. Do designated repetitions and sets.

Task 2   Work on the triceps by extending arms while holding a medicine ball or weighted jugs. In a standing or sitting position, grasp the weighted jugs or medicine ball. Then, raise the arms above the head and flex at the elbow. Raise the object straight up until arms are extended. Do designated repetitions and sets.

Station 2

At this station, students will do tasks 3 and 4. Equipment at this station includes stall bars, mats, ropes, medicine balls, and weight jugs. Students choose the equipment for their particular exercises.

Task 3   Work on the biceps by pulling oneself a designated distance on a mat. Lie at the end of mats that are extended from stall bars. A rope is tied to the bars and extends the length of the mats. In a supine position, pull the body along the mats for a designated distance. Do designated sets.

Task 4   Work on shoulder muscles by abducting the arms along the sides of the body while holding weights in each hand. In a standing or sitting position and keeping the arms straight, raise the arms to desired height and return them to the starting position. Do designated repetitions and sets.

Station 3

At this station the students will do tasks 5 and 6. Equipment at this station will be ropes or tubing, balls, and wasterpaper baskets.

Task 5   Task 5 is performed with a partner. One person removes their shoes. A rope is wrapped around the waist of the second person, whose back is facing the first person. The second person, using legs only, pulls the first person the length of the gym and back. The person being pulled slides their socks along the gym floor.

Task 6   Sit with arms behind the body and used for support. Grasp a ball with the feet. Raise the ball, pivot around, and drop the ball in a wastebasket located behind the participant. Replace the ball and repeat. Do designated number of repetitions and sets.

CONSIDERATIONS FOR YOUNGSTERS WITH DISABILITIES

In this section additional considerations for developing and maintaining the muscular strength and endurance of youngsters with disabilities are presented. The first part of the section deals with considerations applicable to several disabilities and are designated as general, and the second part discusses considerations associated primarily with a specific disability.

As a background to this section it is important to recognize that a disability is so labeled because the condition creates a limitation on how one or more life skills can be accomplished when compared to nondisabled persons. For example, if two levels of a building are separated by stairs, a person in a wheelchair cannot ascend to the second level in that manner. If important information is conveyed through written instructions, a person who is blind cannot obtain the information in that manner. Most things in society are produced for the masses. Thus, the height of handles on weight machines, the weight of barbells, the width of seats on exercise bikes, and the temperature of the air and water in pools are typically designed for nondisabled persons. If someone cannot function using typical modes, they are at a disadvantage. In addition to facility and equipment factors, limitations can also be created by the way programs are conducted. Such factors as the speed at which an exercise is conducted, body position, movement patterns used for an exercise, or the length of recovery time between exercises that a person is given can all create a limitation.

While some limitations may be present, with advances in knowledge and technology, every limitation does not necessarily have to be a barrier. Ramps and elevators enable a person in a wheelchair to get to the second floor of a building, and Braille and auditory recordings help a person who is blind obtain information.

When working with youngsters with a disability, it is important to determine the movement capabilities that they have. Subsequently, when necessary, it is important to make appropriate adjustments for limitations so that they can accomplish desired movement tasks. For example, if an individual has the capabilities to perform a military press to improve the pectoralis and triceps muscles, but cannot do the exercise because of very poor balance, stabilization is a limitation. The participant needs assistance in stabilization so that available abilities to perform the exercise can be used. The information presented in this section emphasizes adjustments that might be appropriate responses to limitations.

General Considerations

While each disability has a particular combination of limitations, there are four limitations that are frequently encountered and are relevant to several disabilities: balance, asymmetry, muscular weakness, and grip.

Balance

The first limitation relates to impaired balance or equilibrium ability. Balance is important in all physical actions, and it is nested in all patterns, whether actions are dynamic or static. If the body is put into an unstable position, it will automatically react to regain equilibrium. This additional movement may make task performance less efficient or impossible to accomplish. These reactions may involve movement of a body part (e.g., an arm, a leg, a hip) to move the center of mass into a more stable position.

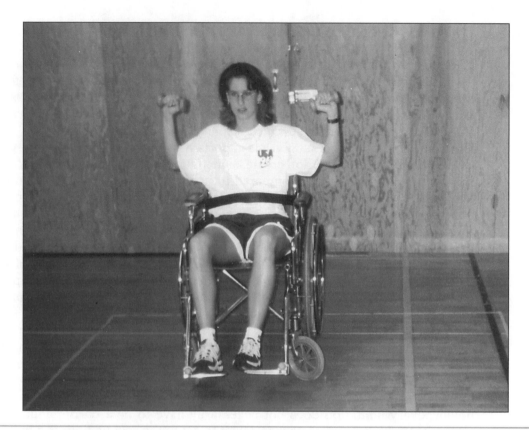

Figure 3.5 Use of strapping to stabilize trunk during exercise

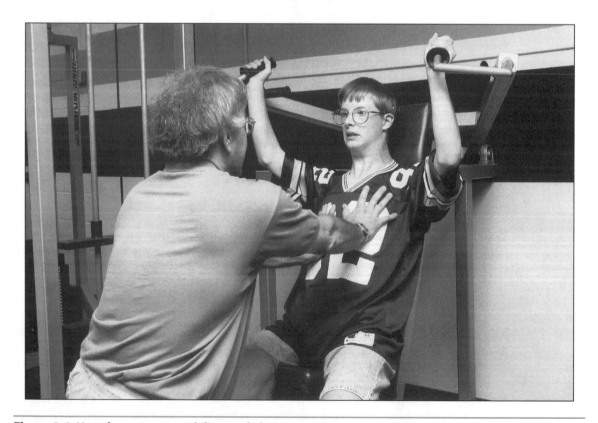

Figure 3.6 Use of a partner to stabilize trunk during exercise

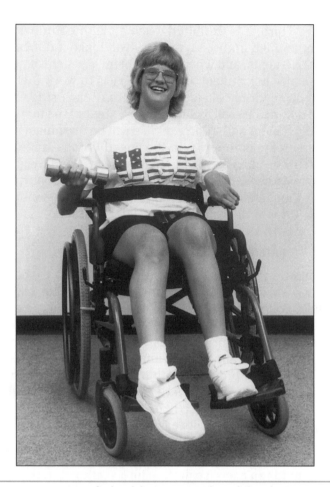

Figure 3.7 Person hangs onto armrest of wheelchair to provide stability during exercise

If equilibrium problems are present, one or more of the following adjustments will usually be very helpful:

• Have exercises performed in the sitting position and use some form of strapping (e.g., safety belts, Velcro straps, trunk binders) to stabilize the trunk (see figure 3.5). If equipment is not available, but staff assistants are present (aides, peer assistants, personal assistants), these individuals can provide physical support (see figure 3.6).

• Another way to adjust to balance problems is to work one side of the body while the other side assists in stabilizing the person. For example, an individual in a wheelchair could hook one arm around the back push handle while pulling or pushing with the other arm. Individuals could hang on to the armrest of a wheelchair (see figure 3.7) or grasp the side of the seat of a chair for support. In a standing position a person could hang onto a wall support, such as a stall bar, while exercising the other side of the body.

Asymmetry

A second limitation that is frequently observed is asymmetry. Asymmetry is present under three conditions. First, it exists when there is an imbalance of muscle strength between one or more body parts on the two sides of the body. Second, it is present when there is a difference in the ROM between similar body parts on the two sides of the body. Third, it is exhibited when a major coordination problem exists between right and left limbs. Asymmetry will make it difficult for the person to do bilateral movements, and when the problem is severe, it could also effect equilibrium. The major adjustment to asymmetry is to work each side of the body independently. Strength imbalances require that each side work against a different load. ROM differences will mean that the extent of the movement and, sometimes, the exact movement path of an exercise will be dissimilar. Incoordination between limbs could create differences in the speed of the exercise, the load that can be controlled, or the movement path that is taken. Hand weights and tubing are good sources of resistance to use since they provide the opportunity to work each side of the body independently. Conditions that most frequently create asymmetry are CP, brain injuries, and progressive muscle disorders.

Muscular Weakness

A third limitation that is frequently present relates to muscular weakness. This limitation is usually created by conditions that create an SCI (e.g., traumatic SCI, spina bifida, polio) and progressive muscle disorders (e.g., muscular dystrophy, multiple sclerosis [MS], Friedreich's Ataxia). Individuals with muscular weakness usually cannot handle normal loads, have a tendency to fatigue very quickly, and may have asymmetry and equilibrium problems as well. Asymmetry and equilibrium were discussed previously, and if present, the same suggestions would apply here. In regard to load, there are additional strategies that can help the individual to some extent. First, it may be most appropriate to use lighter weights. In this regard, lightweight belts can be strapped to a body part. The use of tubing may be most suitable since the minimum load on many weight machines will be quite heavy for many persons with muscular weakness. Another strategy that helps is to divide an exercise motion into sections. For example, the straight-arm lateral raise requires the person to move a load from next to the thigh to above the head. By making this a two-part exercise where the first set has the person move the resistance from the thigh to the midpoint (see figures 3.8a and 3.8b) and the second set is from the midpoint to above the head (see figures 3.8c and 3.8d), the overall intensity of the exercise becomes manageable. This approach not only reduces the duration of the exercise per repetition, but it allows the teacher to adjust the load, if needed, from one set to another. A third useful adjustment is to use gravity-reduced positions. An example would be to have the person perform a biceps curl by placing the arm on a table that is positioned to the side and have the person perform a curl by flexing the elbow and sliding the forearm along the table (see figure 3.9). This will reduce some of the resistance created by gravity that is present when performing the exercise in the normal manner. Another example would be a negative sit-up. The person would sit with knees flexed, feet flat on floor, and arms crossed over chest. The person would slowly lower the trunk to the ground. When the back touches the ground the person would use the arms to help return to the starting position and repeat the exercise.

Fatigue is, of course, associated with muscle weakness. Fatigue may be delayed or minimized by using three adjustments. First, it usually is best to design a program where each muscle is exercised for one to two sets at the most. Secondly, it is helpful to use moderate to slow speeds while exercising as opposed to very fast motions. Third, it is important to provide adequate rest periods. Adequate rest can be assisted by manipulating the order of exercise. After a muscle has been exercised, it is best to work a different part of the body to allow the exercised muscle adequate time to recover before it will assist or stabilize in another exercise.

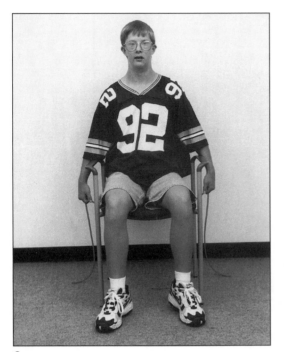
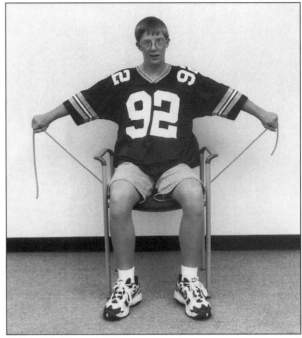

a

b

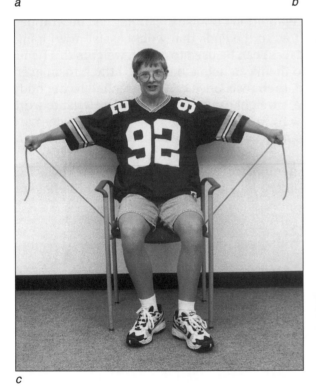
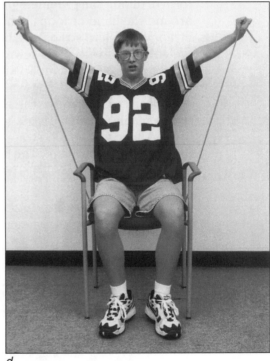

c

d

Figure 3.8a–d Doing an exercise in two parts to provide full ROM while compensating for muscular weakness: (*a*) beginning point for first part, (*b*) ending point for first part, (*c*) beginning point for second part, and (*d*) ending point for second part

Impaired Grip

A fourth limitation that is frequently observed is an impaired ability to grip. This may result from spasticity or severe weakness in the muscles of the hand. Some

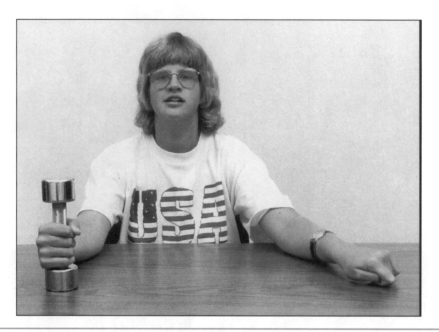

Figure 3.9 Sliding arm across table to overcome the effect of gravity

form of tubing can provide a good adaptation because the tubing can be wrapped around the hand or loops can be tied to the ends that would assist in gripping. Strapping (Velcro straps, ace bandages) can be used to attach weights to a hand. Weight gloves with rings sewn into them can help a person to attach to an exercise bar. If the grip cannot be used, then resistance can be attached to the body part that is to be used. For example, a weight can be attached to the wrist to work the triceps or just above the elbow to work the deltoids. If assistive devices are not available, manual resistance can be used during exercise. Concerning opening the hands to attach strapping or tubing, it is always best not to pull on the fingers to open the hand. The best method would be to push down on the back of the hand (see figure 3.10). This will produce a natural extension of the fingers.

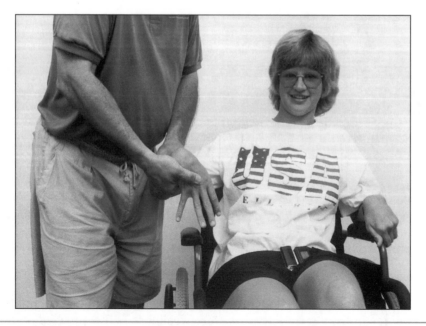

Figure 3.10 Method of safely opening a hand that is affected by spasticity

Even though the extension may not be total, it will be sufficient to allow an attachment.

Specific Considerations

Certain disabilities have relatively specific limitations associated with them that impact on the development and maintenance of muscular strength and endurance. In this section, limitations and their relationship with specific disabilities will be discussed.

Amputation

In terms of the conditioning process, amputation will affect only the limb(s) involved. All other muscles need to be trained as normal. However, amputation can affect balance and leverage, and at times, teachers or program leaders will need to adjust how an exercise is performed due to these factors.

When training, it is important not to ignore the side that has been amputated. The remaining muscles, in the residual limb, need to be kept in balance with the nonaffected side. If there is a bilateral amputation, then the two sides need to be kept in balance. The residual limb(s) can be exercised by attaching weighted resistance to the end of the limb. It is acceptable for the person to exercise while wearing a prosthetic device if the force of the resistance is through the normal axis of the prosthesis. An example would be a bench press where the resistance is pushed by the prosthetic arm or a leg press where the resistance is pushed by the sole of the foot of the prosthetic leg. Thus, the force of the resistance is through the shaft of the prosthetic device. However, if the resistance is perpendicular to the end of the prosthesis, that is, across the shaft, it will be best to do the exercise without the prosthesis. Attaching resistance to the end of the prosthesis when the force is perpendicular could damage the prosthesis and potentially create damage to the residual limb. An example of this type of exercise would be the lateral arm raise to work on the deltoid muscles. If exercise is conducted without a prosthetic device, cuff attachments, tubing, or manual resistance can work well. If there is a single-leg amputation, the individual will have a need to strengthen hip extensor and leg abductor muscles to help maintain a normal gait. If these muscles become weak, the person will most likely use a hip-hiking motion to bring the prosthetic leg forward, which will lead to lower back problems. When a person "hip hikes," the hip on the side of the amputated limb is used to swing the prosthetic leg forward. It is important that the individual regularly strengthen the abdominal muscles and stretch the erector spinae muscles of the lower back to help the muscles in the lower back and hip region adjust to increased strain. If the amputation creates major muscle strength imbalance between two sides, then it would be best to work each side independently.

Progressive Muscular Disorders

This category includes such conditions as muscular dystrophy, MS, and Friedreich's Ataxia. Each specific condition has its own pattern of progression; however, all these conditions make the muscles of the body progressively weaker over time. Because muscles may become weaker regardless of training, the major focus of strength training programs should be to maintain current strength by not allowing weakness to come from disuse and to improve the muscular endurance of the individual so that the effects of fatigue can be reduced. It is very important to ignore the overload principle. Heavy weights (70% of maximum) should never be used. It would be best to use 50% of maximum or less as a resistance. The intensity level is too high if participants do not have their functioning strength and energy level back within 12 hours of a workout. Instructors and participants need to have a good rapport between them so they can freely communicate. If the person is very tired (because of a cold, lack of sleep, energy-taxing day, etc.), the workout should be lightened. It is important not to overwork a person to a point where they become less functional. If this happens on a regular basis the participant will most likely cease exercising rather than be less functional for two days.

In the case of MS, core temperature must be considered. Some individuals with MS become nonfunctional when their core temperature significantly rises. Exercise will naturally produce a rise in core temperature. If a person works at a very high intensity and/or if the ambient temperature is very hot or humid, the core temperature will rise significantly. A person who is susceptible to this condition will become uncoordinated and very, very tired. The teacher should discuss core temperature concerns with persons with MS susceptible to a rise in core temperature. Very hot rooms should be avoided and on extremely hot days workouts should be lessened and/or ways to keep the person cool should be introduced (e.g., frequent fluid intake, wet washcloths to continuously wipe the person down).

Periodically, persons with progressive disorders will go through an exacerbation. This refers to another attack by the disease, which will leave the person less functional. Many times during these periods the person may be hospitalized or absent from a program. After a person experiences an exacerbation, the physical and motor abilities of that person will need to be reassessed and the program adjusted accordingly.

Cerebral Palsy (CP)

There are distinctly different types of CP, but they all produce a motor control problem. Although individuals are not paralyzed, the efficiency of their movement patterns is significantly affected. Because of this, it is very important to assess movement patterns, grip abilities, stabilization abilities, and strength levels on each side of the body. This initial assessment will assist the teacher to best determine the assistance the person will need, the most appropriate exercises for the movement patterns the person possesses, and the best line of pull for each exercise.

While spastic muscles are tight, they are not always strong. If individuals use some of these muscles in ADLs, they could benefit from strengthening these muscles. When spastic muscles are worked, intensity levels above 60% of maximum should be avoided. High-intensity strength work will tend to increase the spasticity for a period of time. In addition, the contralateral muscle group should also be worked to maintain balance in strength.

Individuals with CP will function best if the speed of exercises is kept in a moderate range. Fast speeds tend to create difficulty for persons with CP. If a person's condition creates abnormal postures, then stability problems may exist. Sometimes strapping can help stabilize the body so that an exercise can be performed. Other times, working one side of the body while the other side assists in stabilizing is best. An example is when a person can hook an elbow over a push handle on the back of a wheelchair. The more severe the condition, the more likely that working each side of the body independently works best.

Most individuals with CP will benefit from a 15- to 20-minute warm-up in which static stretching of the muscles to be exercised is used. Persons with spastic CP will have some joints with reduced ROM. While normal ROM may not be restored, it is important to work all exercises through the functional range so that ROM is not reduced.

Spinal Cord Injuries (SCIs)

Traumatic SCI results in the loss of muscle function due to an interruption of neural innervation. All four of the limitations discussed in the general consideration section apply to this disability category. Individuals with an SCI may be paraplegic or quadriplegic. If the person is quadriplegic, impaired sitting balance will be exhibited and will need adjustment. The sitting balance of individuals who are paraplegic will range from minimal control to very good control. The person's balance control during movement definitely needs to be assessed before starting a program. If the person's sitting balance is not well controlled, strapping should be used to provide stabilization.

Individuals in the quadriplegia category most likely will have some impairment in the control of their hands and arms. The use of Velcro straps or ace bandages to attach hands to weights would help. Use of tubing where the tubing can be looped around hands is also helpful. One limitation that is seen in the upper SCI is the inability to contract the triceps, to some extent. Thus, the person either cannot extend the forearm or cannot keep the forearm extended against resistance. Exercises that require an extended forearm position (e.g., lateral raises, flys) will be difficult to accomplish. One method to stabilize the elbow joint is to use air splints. The splints will stabilize the forearm in an extended position and allow the person to work the muscles in the chest and shoulder regions (see figure 3.11).

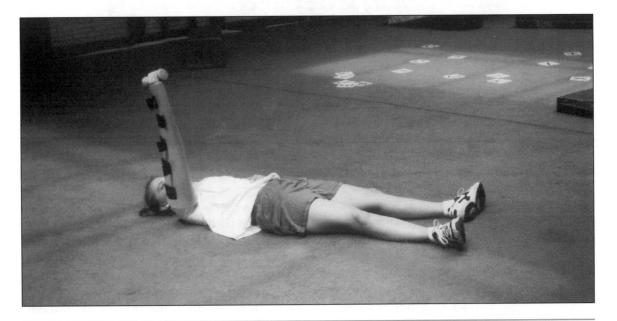

Figure 3.11 Use of splint to stablize arm

Because many individuals who have an SCI function from a wheelchair, many of their postures and actions emphasize flexion. It would be helpful for the person to strengthen the extensor muscles of the body, along with the muscles of the upper back. This will help the person to maintain a more balanced posture and avoid some loss of ROM due to an overuse of flexion muscles.

When working with individuals who have an SCI, there are two important medical concerns that should be understood. The first relates to what is referred to as the tenodesis grip. This is seen in persons who have a cervical-level injury. A

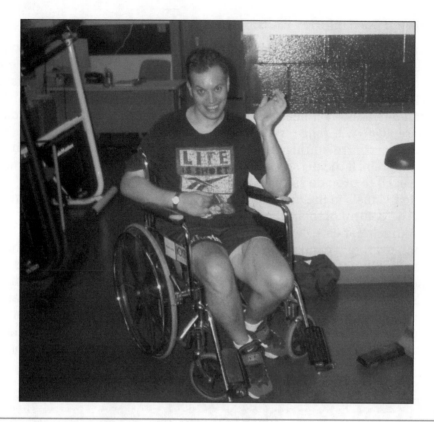

Figure 3.12 Tenodesis grip: fingers tend to flex with wrist extension

natural motion occurs in the fingers when the wrist is flexed and extended. When the wrists are flexed, the fingers extend, and the wrist is extended the fingers flex (see figure 3.12). Physicians and therapists use this natural reaction to help individuals with cervical SCI develop some level of a functional grip. The teacher should never forcefully open the hand by pulling on the fingers. This action could potentially damage the tendons in the fingers and reduce the functional grip that the person possesses.

The second medical concern is known as *autonomic dysreflexia*. This is a serious condition that should receive immediate medical attention when exhibited. The term refers to a reflex response of the autonomic nervous system that results in a total body vasoconstriction. This raises blood pressure and restricts normal blood flow to the working muscles. The vasoconstriction cannot be overcome by the normal compensatory mechanisms of the body. If unabated, the condition could lead to a cerebral hemorrhage or heart failure. This reaction is brought about by a noxious stimulus (often from the bladder or bowel). In many cases a urinary tract infection could trigger this condition.

Symptoms of autonomic dysreflexia include a severe headache, flushed skin above the level of injury, profuse sweating, a fast pulse, and a high blood pressure. Sometimes the reaction is caused by a kink in the person's catheter tubing or a totally full leg bag. If these are present and quickly relieved, the condition may subside. However, if those factors are not present or if the condition does not quickly subside, then emergency medical assistance should be sought.

Most individuals who have an SCI will have incontinence. Incontinence is the medical term for a loss of voluntary control of a person's bowel and/or bladder. There are several different ways that people manage incontinence, and one way is by use of a catheter. A catheter should not impede an individual from engaging in a strength and muscular endurance training program. It would be advisable for the student to empty the leg bag before starting the workout. The reasons for this is that a nearly full bag will bulge at the leg and may sometimes get in the way as the person transfers from one position to another and, secondly, if the attachment from the tubing to the bag should become disconnected, the consequences would be minimal.

A final comment concerning SCI has to do with temperature control. Because the autonomic nervous system adjustments are impaired, people with an SCI do not have the same control mechanisms to manage their temperature as would normally occur. Because the paralyzed muscles lack an ability to shiver to help generate body heat, persons with SCIs cannot adjust to being cold as well as nondisabled persons can. In the opposite situation, where there is a lot of body heat and a need to cool down, the ability to sweat is reduced, and due to the SCI, the individual lacks good vascular control that would shunt the blood close to the skin for conduction of heat. In the environments that strength and muscular endurance training usually take place, the biggest threats come from heat. When the training environment is hot and humid, the student should have a lot of fluids available to drink and their bodies should be kept cool by more frequent rest periods and wet towels to periodically wipe the skin.

Mental Retardation (MR)

Although some youngsters with MR exhibit no decrements in physical fitness, a large majority will show lower physical fitness levels than their peers. Individuals who work with this population may need to be prepared to make adjustments in both performance criteria and methods to meet the needs of these individuals.

When teaching youngsters with MR, it is best to provide small amounts of information at a given time. It is helpful to demonstrate and give lots of cues. Since individuals with MR do not transfer concepts very well, it is important to teach necessary concepts with each exercise/activity.

When working with youngsters with MR, motivation to perform is critical. Most persons with MR will not conceive the big picture. They will not conceptualize the long-term benefits or the need to produce an overload effect. Without understanding those two concepts, most people would not endure the discomfort of training. Most persons with MR will need constant encouragement to work at an intensity/duration level that will produce a training effect. Methods that tend to work well are as follows:

• Ensure frequent success. Progress in small increments. Keep the number of repetitions or trials per set a little lower. For example, do four sets of six repetitions as opposed to three sets of eight repetitons. This makes each set easier to complete, while keeping the volume of work the same.

• Constantly reinforce performance and good effort. Make an effort to be positive. For example, if a person only completes five repetitions, congratulate the student for that effort rather than saying something negative about not doing six. Usually, reinforcement can be social in nature (e.g., praise, smiles, and high fives).

• Reduce the time of formal training workouts. Long, intense workouts will usually produce a period of significant discomfort from fatigue and/or muscle pain. Persons who can envision long-term goals, such as weight loss or greater fitness, and are motivated to achieve those goals will work through the discomfort.

Most individuals with MR have trouble envisioning long-term goals and thus will not be motivated to work through the discomfort of a long, intense workout.

• Make the activity fun. As is true with most youngsters, those with MR are more motivated to work hard in activities that they like. Some youngsters are better motivated when novel elements are employed in or during activity. Examples might be having a person perform push-ups without an object falling off their back, having them listen to music while they are performing an activity, or making an activity part of a game or relay. Sometimes leaders or teachers performing activities with students will help. Giving immediate attainable goals, accompanied with praise, and performing well-liked activities frequently works.

In addition to adjustments for motivation, there are three other factors that may need attention. Many individuals with MR may be less skilled than their nondisabled peers in their movement patterns. It is helpful to use exercises and activities that have simple movement patterns. Youngsters should be provided sufficient time to master movement patterns with very low resistance before increasing the intensity. It helps to constantly cue the person on how to perform the exercise.

Secondly, some individuals with MR exhibit hypotonicity (Davis and Kelso,1982). This means that the amount of tension that can be generated at a given intensity level is less than is observed for their nondisabled peers. Hypotonicity makes exercising more difficult and the onset of fatigue come sooner. There are two adjustments that may help to compensate, to some extent, for hypotonicity. One adjustment is to have longer rest periods between the performance of an activity or exercise. The second adjustment is to have the participant perform fewer repetitions per activity period/sets.

The third factor that needs attention has to do with the potential dislocation at the atlanto-axial joint (atlanto-axial instability) among those with Down's syndrome. This joint is between the first and second vertebrae. A dislocation at this site could create spinal cord damage. It is very important that individuals obtain a medical exam to determine the presence or absence of the condition. If it is present, it is important to discuss with the physician the types of movements and activities that should be avoided. These will usually include activities involving resistance against the head and any extreme flexion of the neck.

GUIDELINES FOR THE DEVELOPMENT OF MUSCULAR STRENGTH AND ENDURANCE

For many years, attention has been given to recommendations regarding frequency, intensity, and duration for the development of physical fitness. For the most part, information regarding exercise prescriptions for the development of physical fitness for adults has been provided and substantiated through research. Most recently attention on physical fitness and physical activity has increased, expanded, and diversified. There have been recommendations regarding (a) the frequency, intensity, and duration of physical activity as well as exercise; (b) physical activity and fitness recommendations for children and adolescents as well as adults; and (c) the development of physical fitness for individuals with disabilities. This section offers guidelines for the development of muscular strength and endurance for youngsters (children and adolescents) with and without disabilities. It is believed that these can be met within the context of the overall recommendations in physical activity presented in chapter 1. However, it must be noted that it may be necessary to modify these overall physical activity recommendations to meet the unique needs of youngsters with disabilities. Guidelines are presented following a review of recommendations in related literature. The final part of this section includes information related to mode and emphasis.

Frequency, Intensity, and Duration

In regard to frequency, intensity, and duration, several recommendations regarding the development of muscular strength and endurance have been offered. Although various individuals and groups have made recommendations, there is considerable agreement regarding the recommendations that have been advanced. The ACSM (1998) presents guidelines for adults and emphasizes that resistance training be progressive in nature, be individualized, and provide a stimulus for all of the major muscle groups. This organization suggests one set of 8 to 10 exercises that conditions the major muscle groups two to three days a week. They go on to recommend that most persons should complete 8 to 12 repetitions of each exercise. This number can be adjusted for older adults and individuals with unique needs.

In a position paper focused on youth resistance training programs, the NSCA (1996), indicates that children should be encouraged to participate in daily physical activity in order to establish good health habits at an early age. Depending on the goal of the training program (i.e., strength or local muscular endurance), this organization recommends one to three sets of 6 to 15 repetitions performed on two to three nonconsecutive days a week for the development of strength and endurance.

Several organizations discussing the need for physical activity for health benefits have recognized the importance of strength and endurance training as an important component of health. These include the ACSM (1995, 1998); the American Heart Association (1992); and the Surgeon General's Report on Physical Activity and Health (U.S. Department of Health and Human Services, 1996). These organizations have recommended performing one set of 8 to 12 repetitions of 8 to 10 exercises two to three times per week for persons under 50 years of age and the same regimen using 10 to 15 repetitions for persons over 50 years of age. Following that review, the President's Council on Physical Fitness and Sports (1996) recommended that strength training programs include 8 to 10 exercises that are performed two to three days per week using one set of 8 to 15 repetitions to fatigue.

In regard to isotonic activities for strength development, Winnick and Short (1985), following their review of literature, recommend that individuals perform 4 to 10 repetitions maximum, three times per exercise session for three to five days per week. In regard to muscular endurance, those authors recommend exercises including light load and high repetitions, following the overload principle. They indicate that the load should be light enough to perform at least 20 repetitions in two to three sets for three to five times per week.

In regard to persons with physical disabilities, recommendations have been made by Lockette and Keyes (1994). Their review of the research indicates that routines of three to nine repetitions would produce the highest increases in strength. They recommend three to five sets of 8 to 20 repetitions for the development of muscular endurance.

Figoni, Lockette, and Surburg (1995) indicate that positive gains in muscle strength and endurance require a minimum of two to three days of resistance training per week with as little as one training session per week for maintenance. They further recommend one day of recovery between days of training. They suggest alternating muscle groups worked or alternating high- and low-intensity training if more frequent training is used. Finally, they recommend more frequent but shorter training sessions for persons with extreme weakness or fatigue.

In regard to the development of strength through isometric exercises, it is recognized that strength gains have occurred as a result of executing isometric exercises at less than maximum intensity. However, from a practical standpoint in implementing programs for youngsters in field situations, maximum contractions are generally recommended because they lead to maximum strength gains and because percent of maximum exertion is difficult to determine (Winnick and Short, 1985). When maximum effort is applied, progression for strength development is inherent in the execution of isometric exercises. Maximum effort is suitable for youngsters both with and without disabilities. Thus, in regard to the development of strength through isometric exercises, Winnick and Short (1985) recommend performance at maximum levels at varying points along the ROM for at least six to eight seconds but not more than 10 seconds. They recommend a frequency of two to three times per day, three to five days per week.

Although isometric contractions develop gains in strength, dynamic exercises are preferred. This is because strength gains through isometric or static contractions are limited to the specific joint angles exercised, and only small improvements in muscular endurance or cardiorespiratory endurance (CRE) occur as a result of isometric training. Also, because of increased blood pressure, isometric contractions may be contraindicated for youngsters with cardiopathic conditions.

Guidelines related to the development of strength and endurance are presented in tables 3.7 and 3.8. These are consistent with the literature in recommending that individuals perform 8 to 10 separate exercises at least twice a week with at least one day of rest in between. It should be emphasized that not all of the 8 to 10 exercises have to be performed in the same exercise session. In fact, it would be preferable not to do this. When using isometric exercises, it is recommended that individuals perform separate exercises two to three times per day, three to five times per week. Again, a total of 8 to 10 separate muscle groups should be exercised at least two times per week. Each isometric contraction should be held for approximately six to eight seconds.

In suggesting guidelines for the development of muscular strength and endurance, it must be emphasized that the overload principle be followed for progress. Generally, it is recommended to exert near maximum muscular tension with relatively few repetitions to develop strength. Lighter weights with greater numbers of repetitions is the best way to develop muscular endurance. In cases where both components are developed, the ACSM (1995) recommends 8 to 12 repetitions per exercise.

When developing and implementing programs for youngsters with disabilities, it may be necessary to modify guidelines. It may be advisable to reduce the number of separate exercises completed per session, which may reduce the number of exercises to be performed each week. It may be necessary to reduce the percentage of maximum effort and/or the number of repetitions of exercises of the same load in regard to strength. Individuals with disabilities may benefit from more frequent exercise/activity sessions of lesser intensity and duration. These modifications are necessary because of factors such as muscular weakness, fatigue, motivation, lower initial levels of fitness, and specific characteristics associated with disabilities. In regard to isometric exercises, the frequency and duration of these does not generally need adjustment for individuals with disabilities. If there is an adjustment, it may be to reduce the number of separate exercises that are included in the total program of the individual. Also, it should be empha-

Table 3.7   Guidelines for Developing Muscular Strength and Endurance Using Dynamic Exercises

General guidelines
Frequency
Perform 8 to 10 separate exercises at least twice per week with at least one day of rest in between.
Intensity and duration
Strength: It is recommended that (a) no load resistance be used initially, (b) load be progressively added as the exercise skill is mastered at each load, and (c) maximum exertions not be encouraged for youngsters, ages 10 to 17. Recommend one set of 8 to 12 repetitions maximum.
Muscular endurance: Perform one set of 12 to 15 repetitions.
Possible modifications for healthy youngsters with disabilities
Frequency
May need to reduce the number of separate exercises completed per session, which may reduce the number of exercises to be performed each week. May benefit from more frequent exercise/activity sessions of lesser intensity and duration.
Intensity and duration
Strength and endurance: May require reduction in intensity to 20 to 50% of maximum repetitions and/or a reduction in duration of activity.

Table 3.8   Guidelines for Developing Strength Using Isometric Exercises

Frequency
Perform separate exercises two to three times per day, three to five times per week. A total of 8 to 10 separate muscle groups should be exercised at least two times per week.
Intensity
Maximum or near maximum effort should be exerted.
Duration
Each contraction should be held six to eight s.

Isometric exercises should be performed at varying points in the ROM.

sized that the recommendations made for persons with disabilities are for those who are otherwise healthy. It is possible that involvement in strength and endurance activities and, in particular, isometric exercise may be contraindicated for certain individuals. This information needs to be determined on the basis of medical consultation.

Mode and Emphasis

There is general agreement that programs designed to develop physical activity may include specific exercises and general physical activities; include a variety of safe and effective training modalities; emphasize activities that are enjoyed; and be a part of well-rounded programs, including those designed to enhance appropriate body composition (BC), CRE, and flexibility/ROM. Decisions about these factors must be personalized and clearly related to objectives and goals associated with programs for youngsters with disabilities.

In their 1998 statement of guidelines, the Council for Physical Education for Children (COPEC, n.d.), indicate that children ages 10 to 12 can develop strength and muscular endurance using formal weight training; however, other activities are generally better suited to the needs of most children. Their guidelines support the use of conditioning exercises using body weight, especially when alternative exercises are offered to allow all children to be successful.

In a position stand, the ACSM (1998) has made recommendations in regard to the nature of a resistance/strength training program for adults that appears to be appropriate for youngsters. In comparing static and dynamic exercises, ACSM recommends dynamic resistance exercises, as they best mimic everyday activities. They also support the use of rhythmical activities performed through a full ROM, with normal breathing patterns during lifting movements. The ACSM statement indicates that although resistance training equipment may provide better feedback to the participant for training purposes, calisthenics and other resistive types of activities can still be effective in improving and maintaining muscular strength and endurance.

The NSCA (1996) has also presented a position paper and literature review on youth resistance training. The NSCA recommends resistance training in youth fitness programs, encourages participation in a variety of sports and activities, and emphasizes the need for age-specific training guidelines.

Writers in the area of physiology of exercise and sport agree about the mode and emphasis of programs designed to develop muscular strength and endurance. Wilmore and Costill (1994), for example, emphasize matching individuals with activities that they enjoy and are willing to continue throughout life. Howley and Franks (1997) believe that strength training can be used as an effective part of an exercise program for children and indicate that health-related goals can be realized by including children in a wide variety of recreational and sport activities.

As mentioned earlier in this section, the mode and emphasis of strength and endurance activities for youngsters with disabilities will need to be individualized and personalized. However, they are very likely to be more alike than different from those of their nondisabled peers. The specific nature of activities will be influenced by the existing abilities of the individual. The emphasis placed on strength and endurance training will be affected by the unique needs of each individual.

Individuals who have a disability frequently have a reduction in their force production capabilities. Most of these individuals would benefit from a strength and muscular endurance training program because it would help them be more healthful in both a physiological and functional sense.

It is the role of the professional leader to be able to help youngsters with disabilities adjust to limitations that are present so that desired training effects can occur. The most frequent adjustments have to do with equilibrium control, asymmetry, significant muscular weakness, and lack of gripping ability. In addition to these adjustments, specific concerns are associated with disabilities, which need to be dealt with for effective implementation of a quality physical fitness program. These include factors that can impact upon frequency, intensity, duration, and the mode of physical activity.

Muscular strength and endurance is most effectively developed by implementing a planned and structured exercise regimen. However, it is highly recommended that participants develop these activities in developmentally appropriate well-liked activities that will lead to a lifetime of involvement.

4

Flexibility/Range of Motion

Paul Surburg

Two terms are used to describe attributes of motion within the body: *range of motion* and *flexibility*. Range of motion (ROM) is associated with the movement or motion within a joint. This term designates the amount of movement a joint may attain in a certain plane or dimension. For example, most individuals without an impairment may bend or flex the wrist to an 80° or 90° angle. ROM is described frequently in degrees of joint movement. In a rehabilitation and conditioning context, ROM may be used to designate the normal amount of motion that should be attained or maintained. Establishing ROM is an early goal of a rehabilitation program.

Flexibility has been defined as structural extensibility, freedom to move, or the maximal amount of movement about a joint. The delineation between flexibility and ROM is not always clear, for ROM has been used to describe flexibility. Anderson and Burke (1991) state that flexibility is the range of motion of a joint and how the joint is affected by parts of the body associated with movement, such as muscles and bones. In this chapter, the term *ROM* will deal with musculoskeletal functioning and the extent of movement within one joint. Flexibility will pertain to the extent of movement possible in multiple joints while performing a functional task. These are the definitions used with the Brockport Physical Fitness Test (BPFT) (Winnick and Short, 1999). Again referring to rehabilitation and conditioning concepts, flexibility is generally an objective of a conditioning or physical fitness program that follows the establishment of normal ROM as part of an adapted physical education program.

ROM and flexibility may be considered part of a health-related flexibility/ROM movement continuum (see figure 4.1). At one end of this continuum is a condition known as ankylosis. This condition describes a joint with no movement, which may be the result of disease, injury, or surgical fixation. This term may describe the status of any joint without movement and is not applied exclusively to the ankle.

The next point along the continuum may be designated as functional flexibility/ROM as described in the BPFT; this represents a clinically acceptable level of

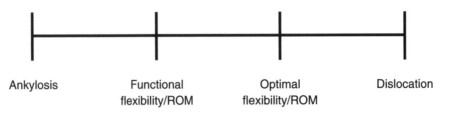

Figure 4.1 Health-related flexibility/ROM continuum

flexibility/ROM that is generally attainable and meets minimal requirements for functional activity. Further along this continuum is optimal ROM. At this point on the movement continuum a person has normal or average movement in a joint (ROM) or joints (flexibility).

The other end of this continuum is dislocation. This condition connotes motion in a joint that is not considered normal. Dislocation of the shoulder (glenohumeral joint), for instance, results in anterior movement normally absent in a shoulder joint. At this point of the continuum, flexibility has been replaced with instability.

In developing a continuum related to flexibility/ROM, another possible designation may reflect an "elite" level of flexibility/ROM. This level may be relevant to participation in physical education activities, including athletics. For example, this level may be important for gymnasts, hurdlers, and swimmers. Although recognized as important for performance, it is not included in the health-related continuum depicted in figure 4.1.

MEASUREMENT OF FLEXIBILITY/ROM ON THE BROCKPORT PHYSICAL FITNESS TEST (BPFT)

Table 4.1 presents test items, areas of the body involved, and a brief description of standards related to flexibility/ROM on the BPFT. In figure 4.2, pictorials of two of 16 joints of the body (right wrist and right elbow extension) using the target stretch test (TST) are presented. Figures 4.3 through 4.6 depict the modified Apley test, the modified Thomas test, the shoulder stretch, and the back-saver sit and reach tests.

JOINT STABILITY

The amount of motion attainable at various joints of the body is predicated upon the nature or structure of a joint. Certain types of joints permit one type of motion, whereas other joints allow two or three types of movement. Table 4.2 provides a brief summary of the different types of joints, amount of movement, and an example of each specific type.

The amount of motion found within two joints of the same type may vary. An example of this motion variation is the ball-and-socket joint of the shoulder (glenohumeral) and hip (femoral acetabular). Part of the potential increase in shoulder movement is a direct function of structural characteristics of this joint. Only 20% of the humeral head is enclosed in the socket (glenoid cavity) of the scapulae. This structural factor accounts for greater mobility and flexibility potential, but this increased movement potential is paid at the price of stability. How many more shoulders have you heard of being dislocated than hips? Joint stability may

Table 4.1 Test Items and Standards Related to Flexibility/ROM on the Brockport Physical Fitness Test

Test item	Body area	Standards
Target stretch test (TST)	ROM of various joints	A score of 2 is a preferred general standard associated with an optimal level of ROM. A score of 1 is a minimal general standard associated with a functional level of ROM.
Modified Apley test	Shoulder flexibility	A score of 3 reflects an optimal level of flexibility/ROM; scores of 2 or 1 reflect functional levels of flexibility/ROM.
Modified Thomas test	Hip flexibility	A score of 3 reflects an optimal level of flexibility/ROM; scores of 2 or 1 reflect functional levels of flexibility/ROM.
Shoulder stretch	Shoulder flexibility	Students attaining a passing score meet a standard associated with an optimal level of flexibility/ROM.
Back-saver sit and reach	Hamstring flexibility	Students attaining a passing score meet a standard associated with an optimal level of flexibility/ROM.

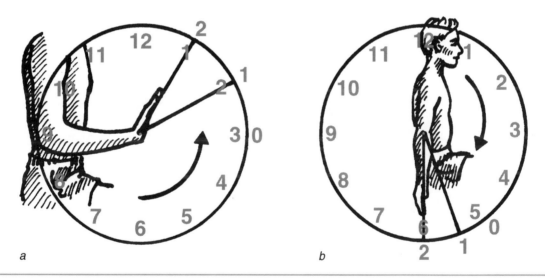

Figure 4.2 Measuring ROM on the target stretch test (*a*) measuring right wrist extension and (*b*) measuring right elbow extension

be affected by the types of exercises that a person uses in a fitness program. Doing deep knee bends, particularly for persons with well-developed leg musculature, may stretch the anterior cruciate ligament and cause instability in the anterior-posterior (sagittal) plane. Along the same lines the traditional hurdler's exercise may stretch the medial collateral ligament and cause knee instability in the lateral plane.

Certain joint-related conditions are predicated upon excessive movement or extensibility of a structure. Persons with hyperextended knees (genu recurvatum)

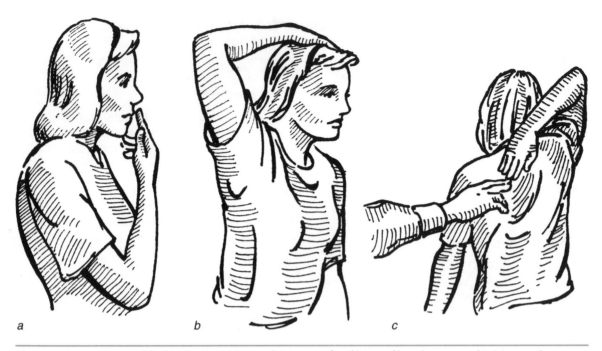

Figure 4.3a–c The modified Apley test: (*a*) mouth—score of 1, (*b*) top of head—score of 2, (*c*) scapula—score of 3

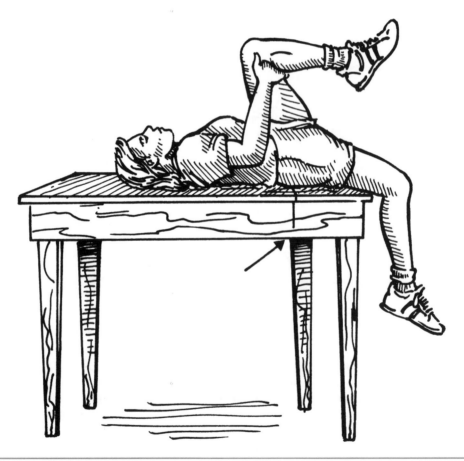

Figure 4.4 The modified Thomas test

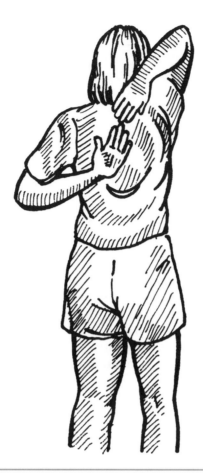

Figure 4.5 The shoulder stretch—right shoulder

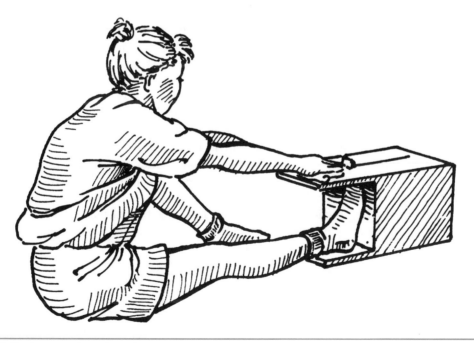

Figure 4.6 Back-saver sit and reach test

Table 4.2 Types of Joint Movement

Type of joint	Movement	Example
Sliding	1	Vertebrae
Pivot	1	Atlanto-axial
Hinge	1	Elbow
Saddle	2	Thumb
Condyloid	2	Wrist
Ball and socket	3	Shoulder

have excessive motion in the sagittal plane. This hypermobile situation is a type of excessive motion that is contraindicated. Stretching of the hamstrings and the gastrocnemius would be counterproductive, for these exercises would increase this hyperextended situation. In this case the physical educator does not want to increase the flexibility of the hamstrings. Development of hamstring strength would be most appropriate for this condition.

DISEASES/CONDITIONS AFFECTING FLEXIBILITY AND ROM

Certain types of disease or conditions will impact upon flexibility/ROM. Neurological disorders, such as upper and lower motor neuron lesions, affect flexibility/ROM. Upper motor neuron diseases, such as cerebral palsy (CP), are characterized by spasticity and hyperactive reflexes. Spasticity is essentially muscle in a state of contraction. This contractile state precludes movement at a joint. Hyperactive reflexes will trigger contraction of muscle when placed in a slightly stretched state. If a person with CP dorsiflexes the ankle too rapidly, the hyperactive reflex may contribute to a contracted or recoil state of the plantar flexors. Certain types of stretching exercises may actually cause this reflex to be initiated with a resultant contraction rather than a stretched or elongated muscle. The teacher should not use any type of bobbing or ballistic stretching with students who have CP because of their hyperactive stretch reflex.

Persons with a lower motor neuron dysfunction, such as polio myelitis or a spinal cord injury (SCI), have muscles that are flaccid and joints with movement limitations potentially due to contractures. Prevention of contractures is important for persons with lower motor neuron lesions (LMNLs) by establishing passive ROM. The physical educator should talk with a physical therapist about the way passive exercise should be done. Issues relating to intensity and duration should be discussed with the therapist.

ROM or flexibility development may not be an objective for certain types of disabilities. Conditions characterized by hypotonicity, such as Down's syndrome, do not need to have flexibility enhanced. For these conditions the focus of a physical fitness program would be to develop strength of various muscle groups with the hope of providing greater stability about body joints. For example, both knee flexor and extensor muscle groups should be part of a strength program. See chapter 3 for additional information on strength development.

GENDER EFFECTS ON FLEXIBILITY

Generalizations are often tenuous at best, but pertaining to flexibility one could state with reasonable certainty that females are more flexible than males. Part of this statement is based upon anatomical differences. Because of the shape of the pelvis, females have greater potential for ROM in the hip region. This difference is evident when comparing the ease with which a female executes a split versus the male. Some developmentalists believe that girls have a greater potential for flexibility development in the trunk area after puberty because of their lower center of gravity and shorter bone length in the legs. While flexibility/ROM in the hip/pelvic region is markedly gender specific, certain joints may not be affected by a gender factor. All the items in the BPFT where gender is considered a factor have separate criterion-referenced health-related standards.

TEMPERATURE INFLUENCE ON FLEXIBILITY

Temperature elevation is an important factor associated with flexibility development. Elevation of tissue temperature is considered a vital step for protecting collagenous tissue. Temperature increments affect the viscoelastic properties of collagen.

Some physiologists contend that heat may influence muscle tone. Lentell et al. (1992) believe that elevation of temperature contributes to flexibility development by reducing alpha motor neuron activity. Reduction in neuron activity causes a type of muscle relaxation and reduced muscle tone. Reduction of target muscle tension is an objective of any flexibility program. Alter (1988) contends that increases in body temperature improve the efficiency of reciprocal innervation. Reciprocal innervation is the reduction in muscle tension of the antagonist muscle and the damping of the stretch reflex while the agonist contracts.

The application of cold and the reduction of tissue temperature is advocated by certain researchers as a method to protect collagenous tissue (Sapega et al., 1981) or optimize plastic deformation of connective tissue. Sapega et al. maintain that heating tissue under low-load stretching conditions and cooling this tissue in a lengthened or stretched position results in a connective tissue deformation of a lasting nature. After certain athletic events, such as after a baseball pitcher has left the game, one often sees the application of ice to the noninjured throwing shoulder as a protective strategy. The only difference between this practice and what Sapega et al. recommend is that the shoulder of the baseball player is not in a stretched position. At the end of a stretching routine, cold could be applied to a target muscle in a stretched position for several minutes.

SETTINGS FOR FLEXIBILITY AND ROM DEVELOPMENT

Flexibility development is considered one of the key elements in a comprehensive physical fitness program, especially for youngsters with certain disabilities. Some physical educators and developmentalists believe flexibility enhancement has been the most neglected of the health-related components of physical fitness.

For individuals with disabilities, flexibility development may be addressed from two perspectives. First, certain joints of the body in many individuals with disabilities have normal ROM. For example, an individual with a paraplegic condition has normal functioning and ROM of upper extremity joints. An aspect of this person's physical fitness program will be to develop suitable flexibility for activities of daily living (ADLs) and for athletic and recreational pursuits involving joints of the body not affected by disability. These persons should strive to attain or maintain optimal levels.

The second perspective deals with joints that have been affected by a person's disability. For example, a person has limited motion at a joint due to arthritic damage and changes. Within the constraints of this situation, flexibility-type exercise may be done to provide some extensibility of the musculotendonous structures. Neurophysiological mechanisms, described in another section, may be the focus of this person's flexibility program. This approach to fitness development should have guidance from medical personnel. Physical educators, however, can and should develop flexibility/ROM of youngsters with and without disabilities in their physical education classes. Physicians and physical therapists should be consulted regarding the scope and limitations of a student's program. Students may strive to attain functional standards associated with the TST or functional levels on the Modified Apley test or Modified Thomas test. The person administering the physical fitness program will utilize this information and personalize this phase of the physical fitness program. Suggestions from support personnel may range from exercises to avoid to suggestions pertaining to neurofacilitation techniques.

REHABILITATION SETTING

A rehabilitation program is often an important phase of a person's medical treatment. The goal of this program is to restore a person with an illness, disease, or injury to an optimal or functional level. Today, rehabilitation programs tend to be rather aggressive, with a person leaving the hospital environment as quickly as possible and restoring a person to a maximal level of functionality.

In the context of physical rehabilitation, an early phase of this program is to regain or reestablish normal ROM in an affected joint or area of the body. A protocol that has served as the gold standard of rehabilitation for persons in adapted physical education involves a progression of movements. This protocol may also be used in educational settings. This protocol consists of four parts: passive movement, active-assisted movement, active movement, and resisted movement. An analysis of this protocol reveals that three of the four stages involve enhancing ROM. As one passively moves a person's body part, the objective of such a procedure is to increase ROM. It should be noted that this is done only if pain is not experienced. The active-assisted phase involves a cooperative endeavor on the part of the individual with a problem or disability and the individual administering the exercise. The individual with a problem or disability tries to reestablish the motion at a joint where there are limitations in movement; the person helping the individual assists in gaining greater ROM. The active phase involves the individual with the problem or disability moving the joint through the full or established ROM without assistance. Resistive movement, the final phase of the four-part progressive sequence, involves progressive increases in resistance during stretching.

Physical fitness programs for persons with disabilities may in essence be part of an individual's rehabilitation program, which may take place not only in the rehabilitation setting but also in the educational setting. Through different means, which will be described subsequently in this chapter, enhancement of joint movement is considered an aspect of a motor or physical fitness program. While these activities are considered part of a fitness program, they are helping to restore or maintain the movement potential of an individual with a disability or problem. Restoration to full or partial potential is rehabilitation. Whether one calls this rehabilitation or the enhancement of physical fitness, the person with a disability is deriving needed benefits through movement and exercise. What greater service can be rendered?

THE EFFECTS OF FLEXIBILITY/ROM ON BODILY CHANGES

An understanding of certain basic concepts of flexibility/ROM development are important to properly improve this component in a physical fitness program. Two distinct components of flexibility development will be discussed in this section of the chapter: collagenous tissue and neurological mechanisms.

Collagenous Tissue Component

Collagenous tissue is a fibrous protein of high tensile strength. This connective material of varying densities and spacial arrangements is found in tendons, ligaments, fascia, aponeurosis, and muscle. Often muscle is thought of as exclusively contractile tissue, but a certain amount of skeletal muscle is comprised of collagenous material. Adhesions, scar tissue, and fibrotic contractures also contain collagen.

When developing flexibility programs for students with disabilities, a teacher does not want to make a joint less stable but, rather, wants to use flexibility exercises to enhance joint motion or structure extensibility. How does a person attain this desired goal and still not compromise joint stability? Part of the answer to this question comes from understanding concepts related to stretching structures with collagenous tissue.

Tissue, such as scar material, and adhesions do limit ROM and flexibility. Individuals with certain disabilities and injuries may have limited ROM because of adhesions or scar tissue. Eliminating or reducing the restrictive effects of these tissues may increase ROM and flexibility. How does one target this type of collagenous tissue without adversely affecting joint stability? The answer, again, depends on understanding the nature of collagenous tissue.

When collagenous tissue is stretched, there is an elongation of elastic elements and viscous elements. Collagen is referred to as viscoelastic tissue. The elastic designation seems most appropriate when discussing stretching and flexibility. A kinesiologist would state that elasticity implies a length change directly related to the amount of applied force or load. The elasticity in collagenous tissue allows a structure to be stretched and to return to its original state. Rubber bands are considered to be elastic, for they may be stretched to a certain point and return to an original configuration or shape. One might think of this example as illustrating a temporary or recoverable elongation. Ligaments and tendons may be stretched, but we hope these structures will assume their original length. Joint integrity is predicated upon the assumption that these structures return to their original length (Surburg, 1981).

Viscous seems to be a strange term to use in a chapter on flexibility. Most persons associate viscous properties or viscosity with fluids and rate of flow. One might think of the viscous element of collagen as a characteristic dealing with resistance to flow or the rate of displacement. The kinesiologist would say that this viscous property is affected by the amount of force applied and the length of time the force is applied, where the rate of displacement or deformation is directly related to the amount of applied force. The model and symbol used to designate a viscous element is the hydraulic piston (see figure 4.7). The velocity of piston displacement is directly proportional to the force. Again, using the rubber band example, if sufficient force is applied over a period of time, there will be a certain amount of displacement without a return to the original condition. There is permanent deformation with this viscous element as opposed to a temporary elongation with the elastic element.

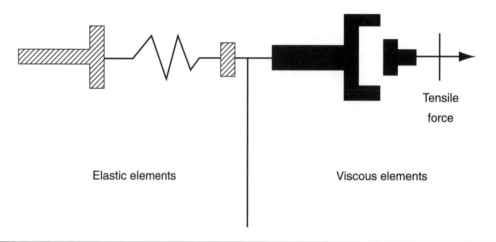

Tensile force

Elastic elements

Viscous elements

Figure 4.7 Collagenous properties

A term sometimes used in lieu of viscous is *plastic*. This term is defined as a linear transformation that remains after the force is removed. Permanent deformation is associated with the viscous element or a type of plastic property as applied to collagenous tissue.

Besides an awareness of the unique characteristics of collagenous tissue, one should be cognizant of the factors that influence the status of these elements. Permanent deformation of the viscous element is enhanced by the application of low loads over an extended period of time. Sapega et al. (1981) contend that to increase permanent deformation, one should elevate tissue temperature during stretching exercises and apply cold before the stretched position or tension is released. For the physical education teacher the practical implications are to make sure tissue temperature is elevated before working on flexibility development. One way that this may be accomplished is by conducting flexibility exercise three quarters of the way through a class period after students have been involved in vigorous activity. The elevation of tissue temperature prior to conducting stretching exercises is a topic that will be addressed in a subsequent section.

Techniques to increase ROM should be designed to produce permanent deformation. Many ROM exercises are oriented toward the viscous element of collagenous tissue. For example, prolonged, low-tension stretching exercises are aimed at affecting the viscous element of this tissue. For the person with CP, attaching a light weight and holding a stretched position for 10 minutes would be a specific application of this concept.

The application of high loads in short periods of time will affect the elastic element of collagen. Stretching exercises incorporating these factors often cause a temporary deformation or elongation. This temporary state may be the exact state a person wants before participating in a sporting event. The wheelchair athlete engaging in a throwing motion may want the extra extensibility for a throwing event but does not need this increment in movement for ADLs. Warm-up exercises emphasizing flexibility would be a way to attain this temporary state.

The concept of stress relaxation is directly related to the characteristics of collagenous tissue. When viscoelastic tissue is stretched and held in a lengthened position, the stress at this lengthened position gradually diminishes. A decrease in tension will occur over a period of time because of the viscous property of collagen. A certain amount of tension is maintained because of the elastic element. Stress relaxation is an underlying principle of certain flexibility protocols. The hold-relax technique of proprioceptive neuromuscular facilitation (PNF) will induce stress relaxation by applying tension to muscular structures during passive tension and isometric contractions. In other words, the tension placed on the muscle in the stretched or contracted state will cause a reduction in tension and increased flexibility. Hold-relax and other PNF techniques will be described in greater detail later in this chapter.

Neurological Component

The second and equally important aspect of flexibility development is the neurological component. Today exercise physiologists and adapted physical educators are keenly aware of the neurological aspects of physical fitness development. For example, the initial stages of strength development, two to six weeks, are neurological in origin rather than affecting the specific muscle tissue. This is one reason why preadolescents exhibit strength changes. Proprioception and kinesthesia, important elements in rehabilitation and conditioning, are basically neurological in nature. As the body of knowledge expands regarding the nuances of flexibility, it is not surprising to discover the vital role that neurological mechanisms contribute to this aspect of fitness.

Two terms will be used as neurological components are discussed. The term *target muscle* refers to the muscle or muscle group that is to be elongated or stretched. Another designation will be the *antagonistic muscle*. This term describes the contralateral, or opposite, muscle or muscle group to the target muscle. If one is stretching the hamstrings, this muscle group is the target muscle; the antagonistic muscle group in relation to the knee is the quadriceps.

A basic premise of flexibility development is to decrease the resistance of the target muscles so that these muscles may be subjected to methods of elongation. One strategy to cause this decrement is to reduce the involvement of the stretch reflex (see figure 4.8). A brief explanation of the stretch reflex should be helpful in understanding the use of certain flexibility techniques and exercises. When a muscle is stretched to a certain extent, receptors in the muscle called muscle spindles are activated. This activation results in an impulse being sent by way of the dorsal root to the spinal cord. At this site a connection is made with a motor effector nerve, and the nerve impulse passes out the ventral root to the muscle. Stimulation of the muscle results in a muscular contraction. The often-heard admonition not to bob or bounce while doing stretching exercises is directed toward not activating the stretch reflex. With bouncing, a person could cause this reflex to be activated, resulting in contraction of the target muscle. In this situation the muscle intended to be stretched instead contracts, which may cause muscle tissue tears rather than developing flexibility. For example, a fast extension

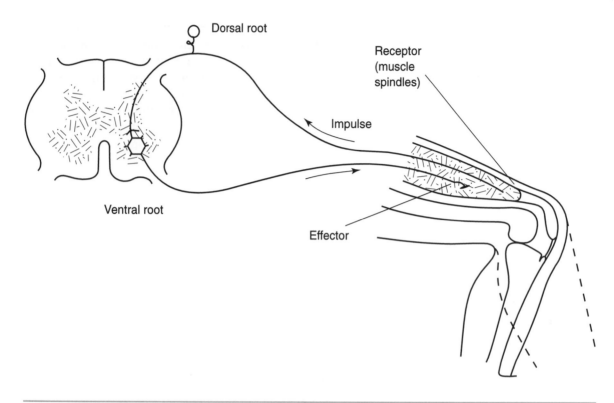

Figure 4.8 Stretch reflex components

of the wrist may cause the wrist flexors to recoil. This recoil is the result of those muscles contracting and could stretch and tear wrist extensor muscle.

Reciprocal inhibition may be used in flexibility exercise routines to reduce the activity of the stretch reflex. This inhibition may be described as damping or reducing the sensitivity of the stretch reflex when executing normal movements. For example, when the elbow is flexed, there is a reciprocal inhibition of the triceps. If this did not occur, a stretch reflex of the triceps would be activated. Certain flexibility protocols, such as PNF, utilize reciprocal inhibition to improve ROM and flexibility.

Reduction of the stretch reflex may be accomplished by other methods, such as the use of cold, massage, and certain relaxation techniques. These three means are common practices with physical therapists and sometimes with adapted physical educators.

A technique called *inverse stretch response* may be implemented to reduce the resistance of the target muscle. The nerve receptor associated with this response is the Golgi tendon organ. This receptor is like the muscle's fuse box. It does not allow the agonistic muscle to contract too forcibly and cause damage to the muscle or bone attachment. If a certain amount of tension is generated and a threshold level is attained in the Golgi tendon organ, the inverse stretch reflex is activated. This reflex causes an inhibition of the contracted muscle, which results in reduced muscular tension. Stretching techniques place the target muscle under tension, which may help to initiate the inverse stretch reflex and cause a reduction in the target muscle tension. For example, the PNF technique of hold-relax or just prolonged static stretching involves an inverse stretch response.

Antagonistic or opposite muscle groups of the target muscle may be involved in a flexibility program. The main strategy with these muscle groups is to develop strength of the antagonistic muscles. Development of strength during the first six to eight weeks is neurological in origin. When a person strengthens both agonistic and antagonistic muscles, particularly with an isotonic regimen, both sets of muscles are elongated. One may interpret this practice as a method of developing a certain functional balance between antagonistic and agonistic muscle groups. For example, developing both wrist flexors and extensors will help wrist flexibility/ROM.

Another way to increase the strength of the antagonist muscles is through facilitation techniques. As noted earlier, PNF techniques will be described in detail in a subsequent section. Several PNF techniques incorporate the concept of *successive induction*. This term refers to contraction of one muscle group followed by contraction of the antagonistic muscles.

There appears to be more involved with the use of PNF techniques for flexibility development than simply the increase in strength of the antagonistic muscle group. Markos (1979) reported a bilateral transfer effect of hamstring flexibility when PNF techniques were used. In her research she found an increase in hamstring flexibility with not only the exercised leg but also with the nonexercised leg. This work illustrates that flexibility development has a distinct neurological basis.

Any flexibility paradigm that portrays flexibility as exclusively the lengthening of connective tissue or the strength development of opposing muscles is an incomplete model. There is a neuro-integration component that must not be neglected. One could say that a person learns flexibility. Learning is used in the context of neurological adjustments or adaptations that allow a person to elongate a muscle for certain movements.

TYPES OF STRETCHING TECHNIQUES

There are various stretching techniques designed to increase flexibility/ROM. In this chapter, techniques to be discussed include passive stretching, active-assisted stretching, active stretching (including static and ballistic stretching), and PNF.

Passive Stretching

As the term denotes, a person is not actively involved in this type of flexibility exercise. An outside force or agent is responsible for increasing joint motion. This agent may be an individual or a machine, such as a continuous ROM machine. At no time during the administration of this exercise do muscles surrounding the joint engage in any type of contraction.

Passive stretching is most often administered as part of a rehabilitation protocol but may be used to help attain goals in an individualized education program (IEP). Individuals are administered this type of exercise because they are very weak, manifest inhibited motion, and/or lack sensation. Passive stretching exercises are generally conducted by personnel with some type of special training in physical rehabilitation or adapted physical education. Regular physical educators should receive guidance from a qualified person with this training, such as adapted physical educators or physical therapists. Some of their guidance will be (1) to support, if possible, the joint to be moved above and below the joint axis; (2) to move the joint in a slow, rhythmic manner; and (3) to elongate structures as far as possible without causing pain. With appropriate guidance and training, physical educators may successfully implement a passive stretching program.

This type of exercise has both advantages and disadvantages for physical fitness enhancement. An advantage is that a partner helps with exercise compliance.

The partner is often able to detect improvements in ROM that the individual with a disability may not be able to discern. Partner-type exercises, in this case with the regular physical educator, promote a spirit of cooperation and concern. In other instances the partner may be a peer. Exercise of any type is usually more enjoyable if done with another person.

Unfortunately, disadvantages are associated with passive stretching exercises. If conducted in an incorrect manner, particularly if done by student partners who extend a joint structure too much, this type of exercise may be painful and harmful. Also, incorrect administration of passive stretching exercises may set off a stretch reflex. For example, moving a body part very rapidly and with a bobbing action would be inappropriate. This could cause a contraction of target muscles rather than an elongation of muscles and create potentially an injurious situation. The key to conducting passive stretching exercises is that the physical educator or adapted physical educator has had proper instruction and training regarding this phase of flexibility/ROM development.

Active-Assisted Stretching

Active-assisted stretching combines efforts of the individual with a disability and a partner assistant, such as an adapted or regular physical educator. This type of flexibility exercise may be conducted in several ways. A traditional method is to ask the individual with a disability to move the joint until movement ceases; then the partner will help move the joint within normal ROM parameters. A variation of the active-assisted routine is to passively move a joint to the end of the ROM and then to have the individual with a disability isometrically contract muscles to hold the joint in this terminal range.

Many of the advantages for partner-type exercise in the passive stretch technique apply to active-assisted stretching exercises. Other advantages are that this technique permits an elongation of muscle not attainable for various disabilities and injuries by other means. This method may help to activate or stimulate weak muscles by stretching the tight antagonistic muscles. Another positive effect may be the establishment of coordinated motor patterns, which is a vital component of the neurological basis for flexibility enhancement.

A disadvantage of this type of exercise is the inability at times of determining the amount of work the individual with a disability is engaging in as the exercise is being implemented. There may be degrees of involvement in the course of several repetitions.

While active-assisted stretching is usually associated with partner exercises, there is another type of assistive exercise. This type of exercise uses gravity to assist in attaining ROM. Stretching the calf muscles by leaning toward a wall is a classic example. For this exercise, gravity provides assistance as the exerciser's body weight moves toward the wall. Potential problems with this exercise will be discussed in the section entitled "Contraindicated Exercises." A main concern is that a person cannot regulate the nature of the movement as well because gravity is assisting in the forward motion toward the wall.

Active Stretching

Active stretching is accomplished by the individual's own efforts without aid of a person or machine. For this type of flexibility exercise, the participant contracts antagonistic muscles and the agonist, or target, muscles are elongated. This type of exercise may not develop as much ROM as active-assisted or passive exercise because the student may not choose to elongate or stretch structures as much as possible.

Specificity of training has a prominent role in the attainment of flexibility. If passive exercises are used, then mainly passive flexibility is developed. Active exercises will enhance active types of flexibility that are needed for ADLs and sport participation. *Total ROM* is a term used to describe a combination of active and passive flexibility. Engaging in strength exercises to increase active ROM is a method used to reduce the disparity between these two kinds of flexibility. Another way to help eliminate this disparity is to have a student engage in functional activities, physical activities, and sports that involve movement of the restricted joint or joints. By working a group of muscles through an ROM, a person is subjecting neuromuscular mechanisms to desired conditions of motion. While one naturally thinks of isotonic strength exercises to help reduce this disparity zone, there is evidence (Hardy, 1985) that longer periods of isometric exercises will also help. This is especially true of PNF exercises, which will be discussed later on in this chapter.

Static

Active flexibility exercises may be placed into two categories: static and ballistic. Static stretching consists of slowly elongating muscle and related structures until further movement is markedly limited and accompanied by discomfort. Generally this position is maintained for a period of time. Over time there appears to be reduction in tension and a partial relaxation of the target muscle. The actual duration of stretch may vary from six seconds to 45 minutes. Longer periods of stretching, often called "prolonged stretching," should be done with low forces or loads. It has been recommended, for example, to use between 3 and 5% of body weight as a guide for the amount of poundage used to provide a stretching force for prolonged stretching exercises (Lentell et al., 1992).

Static stretching is considered more appropriate than ballistic stretching for persons with and without disabilities. Static stretching requires less energy, results in less injury, and may help to reduce muscle soreness. Sitting with the knee extended and pulling slowly on a towel that is around the bottom of the feet is an example of static stretching of the calf muscles.

Ballistic

Ballistic stretching is often described as a momentum exercise. A person bounces, twists, and swings a part of the body to lengthen muscles and associated structures. This type of stretching technique is generally not recommended for most individuals and is contraindicated for persons with many types of disabilities. Reasons cited for not using ballistic stretching are (1) the stretch reflex may be activated and muscle tissue may be damaged, (2) angular momentum of the body cannot be adequately controlled, and (3) neurological adaptations are not likely to develop.

One reason people do ballistic stretching is that many sport and physical activities are ballistic in nature. While this is an irrefutable fact, there are other ways to develop or train muscles for the ballistic nature of sporting activities. One of the most common ways is the actual practice of the athletic event. Considering the possible problems and damage that may result from ballistic stretching, one should avoid this type of exercise for physical fitness development.

Proprioceptive Neuromuscular Facilitation (PNF)

PNF is a system of exercises designed to help develop strength, flexibility, coordination, and kinesthesia. This regimen of exercises was developed by physician Herman Kabot and refined by physical therapists Margaret Knott and Dorothy Voss. The focus of this section will be on the development of flexibility and ROM through PNF techniques.

PNF is based upon four neurophysiological concepts: reflexes, resistance, irradiation, and successive induction. Reflexes may be used to enhance motion for strength development. In the case of flexibility development, diminishing the effect of the stretch reflex is a goal of a flexibility program, as explained in an earlier section, and may be accomplished through PNF techniques. Resistance may be used to develop the strength of contralateral muscles or promote types of neurological activity, such as reciprocal inhibition. Irradiation deals with spread of excitation to surrounding muscles. For flexibility, irradiation may involve exciting and then diminishing muscle activity in surrounding muscles prior to stretching a muscle group. Successive induction is the contraction of one set of muscles followed by the contraction or activation of an antagonist muscle group. For example, a person contracts the hip flexors and then the hip extensors. Related to successive induction is reciprocal inhibition, which is a useful neurological mechanism for flexibility development because the stretch reflex is diminished or eliminated. With reciprocal inhibition in operation, the agonistic muscle contracts without the stretch reflex of the antagonistic muscle coming into play and creating tension in the antagonistic muscle. In essence, the facilitation and inhibition of neuromuscular activity is an objective of PNF techniques. There are at least nine PNF techniques used by persons involved with rehabilitation and conditioning to develop strength, flexibility, and other physiological attributes. Of these nine, five techniques are used to enhance ROM or flexibility. Each is discussed in the following paragraphs.

Rhythmic Stabilization

This technique involves an isometric contraction of the agonistic muscle group followed by an isometric contraction of the antagonistic muscle groups. This alternate contraction of agonistic (target muscle) and antagonistic muscle groups is done with the idea of gradually increasing the ROM as one changes the positions of a student's limb. The increase in motion may be evident during one exercise session or over a series of sessions.

This and other techniques may be administered in two different ways. Individuals with specialized training in PNF use these techniques with diagonal, spiral patterns. These patterns involve an intricate set of movements that a person must learn through specialized training. Advocates of PNF contend that these diagonal patterns elicit irradiation, which helps to facilitate muscle functioning. It should be noted that many sporting and recreational activities, as well as ADLs, involve movements in diagonal patterns rather than motion in a cardinal plane. A key ingredient in PNF patterning is that both the participant and the assistant must understand all the movements of the diagonal, spiral patterns. Explanations of these patterns are found in several books (Voss, Ionta, and Myers, 1985; Hollis, 1981) and are beyond the scope of this book.

An alternate method of executing these techniques is to execute movements in the cardinal planes. This method is recommended for the physical educator. For example, to work on shoulder flexibility a person would do abduction and adduction movements in the frontal plane. Initially, a person would abduct the arm until

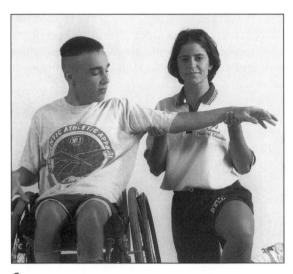
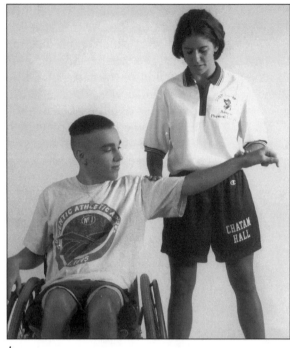

a

b

Figure 4.9a–b Rhythmic stabilization—a PNF technique: (*a*) resistance to adduction and (*b*) resistance to abduction

there is no motion. Then an assistant would apply pressure at or above the elbow so that the participant engages in an isometric contraction. This is followed by an isometric contraction of the shoulder abductors (see figure 4.9a–b). The arm is now slightly more abducted and another abducted isometric contraction is performed. As the alternate contractions are done, increased ROM is hopefully attained. To increase hamstring ROM, this technique would be done in the sagittal (anterior-posterior) plane.

For the student who has trouble successfully executing the modified Apley test in the BPFT, rhythmic stabilization of the abductor/adductor muscles of the shoulder will help the abduction movement of this test. Rhythmic stabilization could also be used for the external rotation phase of this test. With improvement in flexibility, a student can more readily comb the hair on the back of his/her head as well as score better on the modified Apley test.

Hold-Relax

This technique involves a teacher passively moving an extremity as far as possible into a position with the target muscles in an elongated or stretched position. Next, the student contracts the target muscles while the teacher applies sufficient resistance to cause an isometric contraction. After a six-second isometric contraction of the target muscle, the teacher has the student relax the target muscle and places the target muscle group into an elongated position. This is followed by another isometric contraction of the target muscle group. This sequence may be repeated several times with, hopefully, increased ROM and change in joint angle.

An example for improving hamstring flexibility will be given using the hold-relax technique applying the cardinal plane approach. The student assumes a back-lying position, and a passive straight leg lift is done by the teacher through as much ROM as possible. With the leg in a flexed position at the hip and the knee extended to a point of mild discomfort, the student is told to extend the leg at the hip with the teacher applying sufficient forward pressure to enact an isometric contraction of the student's hip extensors (hamstrings). After a six-second isometric contraction, the student relaxes the target muscles. The teacher initiates the exercise again by passively bringing the leg into a deep stretched position. This is followed by an isometric contraction of the hip extensors. This procedure may be repeated several times with hopefully more hip flexion as the exercise is repeated (see figure 4.10a–b).

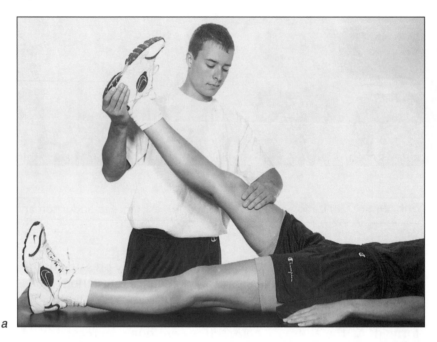

a

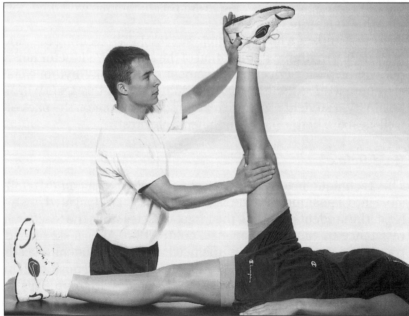

b

Figure 4.10a–b Hold-relax —a PNF technique: (*a*) passive movement of hip flexors and (*b*) isometric contraction of hip extensors

Contract-Relax

This technique, contract-relax, involves a maximal isotonic contraction of the target muscle groups after these muscles have been put passively on maximal stretch. In essence, this technique is similar to hold-relax except the contraction of the target muscle groups is an isotonic rather than an isometric contraction. This example is done in the cardinal plane. A student assumes a back-lying position, and a passive straight leg lift is done by the physical education teacher. With the leg in a flexed position at the hip and the knee extended, the student is told to extend the leg at the hip. The teacher applies forward resistance while the student isotonically contracts the hip extensors. This sequence may be repeated five or six times.

Hold-Relax-Contract

This PNF technique has been called an active technique by Hardy (1985). The term *hold* in any PNF technique refers to an isometric concentration. Hold-relax-contract is essentially the hold-relax technique described earlier with one additional component. After the isometric contraction of the target muscle, the student actively contracts the antagonistic muscle group, but no resistance is provided by the teacher. For example, when working on the flexibility of the hamstrings and after the isometric contraction of the hamstrings, the student would isotonically contract the hip flexors and elongate the hamstrings. Research by Hardy (1985) has shown this technique to be more effective than hold-relax.

Contract-Relax-Contract

This is another of the "active" techniques. Contract-relax-contract is similar to or a continuation of contract-relax. After a student has finished isotonically contracting the target muscle group, the student then isotonically contracts the antagonistic muscle, but the teacher does not apply any resistance. This technique has been used more frequently in the last decade to enhance flexibility development (Surburg and Schrader, 1997).

If the objective is to work on back muscle flexibility, the protocol would be as follows. A student would assume a sitting position with the legs in an extended position. The teacher would passively move the upper part of the body into a flexed or curled position. The student would then extend or straighten out the back as the teacher provides resistance to the student's isotonic contraction of the back muscles. Following this contraction, the student then actively curls the back muscles by contracting the abdominal muscles. This sequence may be repeated five or six times.

THE RELATIONSHIP OF STRENGTH AND FLEXIBILITY DEVELOPMENT

Many people do not think of strength development as a form of flexibility exercise. Ironically, overdevelopment of strength has been associated with the idea of a muscle-bound person. The idea that strength development may reduce flexibility is totally incorrect. The only possible way that incorrect strength regimens may affect functionality is the establishment of an imbalance in strength between agonists and antagonists or not exercising throughout the ROM.

Two key factors must be considered when viewing strength development from a flexibility perspective. First, a person should do a strength exercise through the full ROM for both agonist and antagonist. This type of protocol insures not only a balance of strength development but also that both groups of muscles (agonist and antagonist) may be elongated through their normal ROM. For example, as a person does an elbow curl, the tricep is placed in a stretched position. When the triceps extends the elbow, the biceps is elongated.

The second use of strength exercises for flexibility development involves eccentric contractions, or negative work. This type of exercise not only develops a type of strength, but the muscle is stretched while contracting. During eccentric contractions the number of contractible components decrease with a concomitant increase in tension. This increase in tension and stress results in greater elongation of the respective structures, which may facilitate flexibility development. The eccentric development of muscles on the lateral side of the ankle (peroneal muscles) may help reduce the possibility of a person spraining an ankle when he/she twists (inverts) the lateral side of this joint.

TECHNIQUES TO REDUCE MUSCLE TENSION

Decreasing the tension in a muscle is a key factor in flexibility development, particularly with certain types of disabilities, such as spastic CP. As noted in an earlier section, reduction of the stretch reflex is a key neurophysiological mechanism in the enhancement of flexibility. This reduction of reflex activity may be subsumed under the classification of relaxation strategies. Strategies or methods of attaining muscle relaxation may be considered as indirect or direct approaches to flexibility development.

Indirect methods attempt to relax target muscles through nonexercise means. Some of these methods are a precursor to some types of flexibility protocol. A method that transcends decades of time is the application of heat to help relieve pain, reduce muscle tension, and make structures more supple for flexibility exercises. Hot packs, whirlpools, heating pads, and Jacuzzi are a few examples of applying heat for muscle relaxation. In physical education, a heated swimming pool may be used to help relax the muscles.

Another indirect method is the use of cold, often referred to as *cryotherapy* in sports medicine. Cold seems to desensitize stretch receptors and possibly blocks receptor excitability. A precaution regarding the use of cold is the possibility of causing frostbite in an isolated area of tissue. When comparisons are made between the use of heat or cold to enhance flexibility, heat usually seems to be the more effective modality.

Direct methods involve specifically designed exercises to reduce muscle involvement or tension. PNF includes exercises that attempt to reduce the tension of target muscles by initiating neuromuscular mechanisms, such as reciprocal inhibition and inverse stretch response.

Another direct technique to reduce muscle tension involves the use of relaxation techniques. Progressive relaxation exercises developed by Jacobson (1938) attempt to voluntarily relax skeletal muscles. A person maximally contracts a muscle group and then relaxes this muscle group. The individual contracts the muscle group at half the maximum effect and then relaxes the muscle group. This is followed by additional diminished contractions and subsequent relaxation.

Relaxation responses were investigated and popularized by Benson (1980) of the Harvard Medical School. This physician identified four elements necessary to create a relaxation response. These elements are a quiet environment, a mental set, a passive attitude, and a comfortable position. For an extensive coverage of this relaxation technique, consult his book, entitled *The Relaxation Response* (Benson, 1980).

Most indirect methods are not viable options for teachers of physical education providing opportunities for persons with disabilities to enhance their physical fitness. The school physical therapist may use indirect methods for developing flexibility/ROM. The direct methods, however, are options for all persons involved in facilitating physical fitness for individuals with disabilities. The use of warm water in a swimming pool, PNF techniques, and relaxation protocols are recommended methods available for physical education teachers.

GUIDELINES FOR IMPLEMENTING FLEXIBILITY/ROM EXERCISES

As a physical education teacher embarks on developing an ROM/flexibility program for a student with a disability, the individualized nature of the program is a foregone conclusion. There are, however, general guidelines that teachers should follow as individualized programs are implemented.

Warm-up and Cool-down

Most persons who are involved in any type of physical activity are familiar with the term *warm-up*. There are several types of warm-ups. The familiar concept of warm-up involves engaging in certain exercises and motions before starting to participate in some type of physical activity (Smith, 1991). This type of warm-up may be categorized into general and specific exercises. General warm-up consists of a series of movements and exercises that are not directly related to the soon to be engaged in activity. A person may do jumping jacks and running in place before engaging in physical fitness activities. Some of these exercises usually include stretching, in some manner, muscles of locomotion and upper extremity muscle groups. According to physiologists, general warm-up exercises are intended to increase muscle and core temperature (McArdle, Katch, and Katch, 1991). For certain individuals, the psychological benefits are as important as the physiological benefits. If a person believes he or she cannot engage in physical activity without warm-up then there is definitely a psychological element to warm-up. There is experimental evidence showing that warm-up has a large psychological element (Massey, Johnson, and Kramer, 1961).

The second type of warm-up is referred to as specific warm-up. An individual engages in exercises and movements that are directly related to the activity of choice. For example, a wheelchair tennis player will swing his racket in motions to replicate the forehand, backhand, and serve. Initially these motions may be done at half speed, and with each replication of a tennis stroke the velocity is increased.

Another type of warm-up exercise is intended to elevate the body temperature prior to engaging in a specific set of flexibility exercises. A person may jog for a period of time or ride a bicycle before doing flexibility exercises for the legs. The intent of this type of warm-up exercise is to influence the viscous properties of collagenous tissue. It is an established fact that there is an inverse relationship between temperature elevation and viscosity.

A practical way to elevate tissue temperature is to have individuals engage in vigorous activity and then devote a certain amount of time to specific flexibility protocols while the body is in this elevated temperature state. This approach is illustrated in table 4.3. For some disabilities this temperature elevation may be assisted by doing exercises and activities in a heated pool. This approach may be particularly helpful for individuals with spasticity and certain types of contractures.

Table 4.3   Implementing Flexibility Concepts in an Activity Session

Application	Explanation
Phase I Engage in pre-exercise warm-up (five min).	Students are used to having a warm-up period. This phase has both physiological and psychological benefits.
Phase II Engage in activities of the physical education unit (25 min).	A well-planned and diverse program of activities is important for students with and without disabilities.
Phase III Engage in PNF techniques such as contract-relax to work on flexibility (five min).	Involving students in specific flexibility activities with an elevation in tissue temperature will protect the collagenous tissue of muscle and ligaments. Using contract-relax will involve certain neurological mechanisms to enhance flexibility.
Phase IV The class will participate in some cool-down activities at the end of the period (five min).	These activities will help the body make a transition to a less active state.

As important as warm-up is prior to engaging in physical activities or flexibility exercises, cool-down or warm-down is an essential element of an activity program. The cool-down phase assists body mechanisms in adjusting from an active phase to a resting phase. The objective of this phase is to reduce the potential for muscle soreness and to facilitate the removal of waste products. Some individuals believe that stretching exercises should be part of the cool-down protocol. Table 4.4 applies warm-up and cool-down recommendations as well as other concepts in an activity session.

Frequency, Intensity, Duration, and Mode

Programs for students with disabilities must be truly individualized to obtain the greatest benefits of all types of physical fitness activities, including flexibility exercises. General guidelines and modifications for use with youngsters with and without disabilities are presented in this section and are summarized in table 4.4. When applying these guidelines, it should be emphasized that they be carried out in accord with recommendations for daily activity or near daily activity.

In regard to frequency, it is recommended that youngsters experience daily involvement in physical activity. If specific exercises are used for the development of flexibility/ROM, it is recommended that they be conducted at least three days per week. The intensity of exercise should be a stretch to a position of mild discomfort while engaged in specific exercises and no discomfort while engaged in general physical activities.

Table 4.4 Guidelines for Achieving Flexibility

General guidelines
Frequency
At least three days per week when using specific exercises; daily involvement in general physical activities.
Intensity
To a position of mild discomfort while performing specific flexibility exercises; no discomfort when engaging in general physical activities.
Duration
During flexibility exercise, three to five stretches of 10 to 30 s for each stretch; during general physical activities, stretches should be held in accord with fitness levels.

Possible modifications for healthy adolescents with disabilities
Frequency
Ranges from three days per week to two to three times daily in formal exercise programs; daily involvement in functional daily physical activities. Overall, exercise sessions may need to be conducted more frequently for longer durations.
Intensity
No change
Duration
For persons with unique needs, fewer repetitions of longer stretches may be most appropriate during exercise sessions. When exercising, the duration of stretches may range from one s to 10 min; three to five repetitions of stretches not exceeding 30 s may be appropriate; long stretches may be limited to one repetition.

The guidelines presented in table 4.4 in regard to frequency and intensity are in accord with recommendations in the literature. In their guidelines for achieving and maintaining flexibility for adults, the ACSM (1998) recommends a minimum frequency of two to three days per week and at least four repetitions per muscle group. In their 1998 guidelines related to the physical activity of children, COPEC (n.d.) indicates that some regular stretching for children ages 10 to 12 is appropriate either in the form of age-appropriate flexibility exercises or activities that promote flexibility, such as tumbling and stunts. Following their review of literature, Corbin and Noble (1980) indicate that most programs recommend stretching several times daily. Alter (1988) recommends stretching once a day for the maintenance of flexibility. Lockette and Keyes (1994), in making recommendations regarding individuals with disabilities, indicate that stretching exercises need to be performed at least three times a week to maintain flexibility. Following their review of literature, Winnick and Short (1985) encourage daily involvement in flexibility training, with exercises performed two to three times per day in programs for youngsters with disabilities.

In regard to intensity, the ACSM (1995, 1998) supports stretching to a position of mild discomfort for healthy adults. Corbin and Noble (1980) conclude that stretching must exceed normal length to be effective. Lockette and Keyes (1994) recommend no pain and only slight tension that slowly diminishes with the stretch. They recommend beginning stretching for 10 seconds and then increasing time and intensity according to the tightness of the muscle group. Winnick and Short (1985) indicate that stretching should not exceed 10% of the current flexibility/ROM of the individual.

When implementing programs, it must be remembered that the intensity of flexibility exercises is related to the type of exercise (active versus passive) and the condition of the student. There must be a degree of elongation or stretching to affect the collagenous tissue. With the execution of a flexibility exercise, a certain amount of discomfort may be experienced. In a physical education setting, this discomfort should not graduate into ongoing encounters with pain by the student. Another technique is called passive, prolonged stretching. A light weight between 5 and 10 pounds (Irrgang, 1994) or 5% of a student's body weight (Lentell et al., 1992) is attached to a limb to help keep target muscles in a stretched position. This stretched position is maintained for 10 to 15 minutes. With any type of flexibility/ROM exercise the intensity of the specific exercise should not cause discomfort beyond a mild sensation. When general physical activities are engaged in to improve or maintain flexibility/ROM, no discomfort is recommended.

The duration of a stretching exercise is often cited in the literature as 6 to 12 seconds (Corbin and Noble, 1980; Alter, 1988). Bates (1971) maintains that up to 60 seconds may be needed to maintain or increase flexibility. The ACSM (1995, 1998) recommends a duration of 10 to 30 seconds for each stretch in programs for healthy adults. Lockette and Keyes (1994) recommend stretches for 10 to 60 seconds when working with persons with physical disabilities. They also support stretches for longer periods of time after workouts (during cool-down) to increase ROM and decrease muscle soreness. Lasko and Knopf (1988) recommend 30 to 60 seconds of active, slow stretching in a book oriented for persons with disabilities. These longer durations of time definitely involve a low-load, prolonged stretch type of exercise. When engaging in physical activities to improve flexibility/ROM, a holistic approach should be addressed. One must consider the status of all health and fitness factors in determining the duration of involvement in physical activities.

Some sports medicine authorities believe the entire flexibility program should last no longer than 10 minutes (American Academy of Orthopaedic Surgeons, 1991). The number of exercise repetitions within an exercise session varies: three (Winnick and Short, 1985), 5 to 15 (Alter, 1988), and 5 to 10 (Irrgang, 1994). In the final analysis the number of repetitions is determined by the objectives and goals of the program and how well a student is responding and benefitting from the specific type of flexibility exercise.

In regard to type or mode of exercise, there is agreement that youngsters benefit from formal exercises, general physical education activities, and ADLs as they develop flexibility/ROM. Also, static, dynamic, and PNF techniques enhance flexibility/ROM. In regard to types of stretching, the ACSM (1998) recommends a general stretching program that exercises the major muscle tendon groups using static, ballistic, or modified PNF (contract-relax, hold-relax, active-assisted) techniques. Following their review of literature, Winnick and Short (1985) state that static stretching has been more highly recommended than ballistic stretching for beginners and those not training for sport competition. In regard to types of stretch, they suggest that if ballistic stretching is used, it should be preceded by warm-up consisting of static stretching. Lockette and Keyes (1994) strongly favor static versus bounce-type stretching exercises for persons with physical disabilities, since bouncing can tear tissues or cause injuries in other affected areas. Surburg (1995) recommends avoiding ballistic exercises for persons with physical disabilities even for sport and ADLs, since flexibility/ROM can be developed while performing or practicing these activities themselves. Lockette and Keyes (1994) and Surburg (1995) feel that dynamic stretching should not be used for stretching spastic muscles. In conclusion, static, PNF, and nonbounce-type dynamic exercises are recommended herein for the development of flexibility/ROM for youngsters with disabilities.

General Activities to Develop Flexibility/ROM

This chapter focuses on the use of exercise to enhance flexibility/ROM. This is appropriate, since exercises may be selected and designed to efficiently enhance flexibility/ROM. Also, the principles underlying flexibility/ROM development are effectively explained and demonstrated using exercise. However, it is critical to recognize that continual involvement in games, sport, aquatic and rhythmic activities, dance, and other physical activities is as, if not more, important than exercises for the development of flexibility/ROM, particularly in the context of health-related physical fitness. As explained in chapter 1, involvement in physical activity is the foundation for the development of health-related physical fitness and is enhanced when activity brings success and is enjoyed. Offering broad-based programs to youngsters increases the likelihood that they will be engaged in physical activity—in both childhood and in adulthood—more frequently, with more intensity, and for longer periods. For example, youngsters riding horseback may potentially impact on lower extremity flexibility to a greater extent than those involved in more "sterile" exercises. Individuals who enjoy archery or fencing may develop upper body flexibility to an extent greater than if they simply engage in formal exercise, since they are more likely to be included more often, more intently, and for longer periods of time in these activities. The key to programming for health-related goals is to personalize involvement in physical activity. Communication with youngsters and providing opportunities for choices enhances success, participation, and health-related benefits.

Involvement in many gross motor activities will involve and possibly nurture flexibility. This includes participation in ADLs, in physical recreation activities, and in athletics. Different activities, however, involve different regions of the body to a different degree. Activities can be analyzed in regard to involvement and contribution to flexibility management. A sample of physical activities utilized for the development of flexibility is presented in table 4.5 and figures 4.11 and 4.12.

Positioning of Persons

An important consideration when involving a person in flexibility routines is the initial positioning of the student. Initial positioning takes on added significance when working with persons who have disabilities. Positions may (1) influence or control the effect of gravity; (2) reduce potential injury; and (3) diminish adverse reactions of certain types of disabilities, such as hyperreflexive muscle action of persons with CP. Gravity may have a particularly profound impact on flexibility exercises. Bobbing types of movements that use the effect of gravity on body movements may trigger the stretch reflex, which may cause injury. Activation of the stretch reflex applies not only to students with CP but persons with no neurological involvement.

Table 4.5   A Sample of Physical Education Activities for the Development of Flexibility/ROM

Activity	Area developed
Horseback riding	Lower body flexibility
Archery	Upper body flexibility
Rowing, canoeing, kayaking	Upper body flexibility
Bowling	Upper and lower extremity flexibility
Bicycling	Lower body flexibility
Dancing	Total body flexibility
Golf	Trunk and shoulder flexibility
Stunts and tumbling	Total body flexibility
Wrestling	Total body flexibility
Table tennis, tennis, racquetball, handball	Total body flexibility
Swimming	Total body flexibility
Alpine skiing	Lower body and trunk flexibility
Fencing	Upper body flexibility
Rock climbing	Total body flexibility
Sledge hockey	Upper body flexibility
Frisbee	Upper body flexibility
Fishing	Upper body flexibility

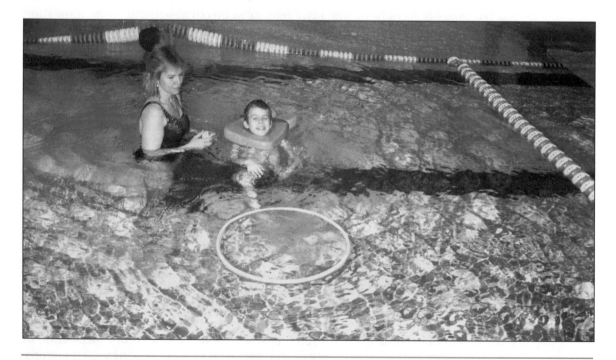

Figure 4.11 Swimming: a fun way to stimulate flexibility/ROM

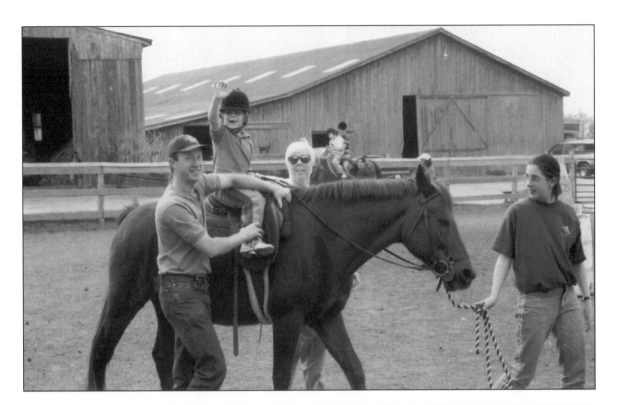

Figure 4.12 A youngster with cerebral palsy riding horseback

In certain positions, a bobbing effect may become more intense because of a gravitational effect. For example, a person in a standing position attempting to stretch the back and hamstring muscles by touching the toes may tend to do bobbing types of movements because gravity is assisting in the exertion of the toe-touch (see figure 4.13a). If one begins this exercise in a straight leg sitting position, control of the toe-touching movement is more likely, for the intended motion is not as readily aided by gravity. Yet, there is some concern that executing a toe-touch from a sitting position may put too much stress on the vertebrae (see figure 4.13b). This concern may be resolved by assuming this position with only one leg extended. To reduce the effect of gravity and gain more control over the movement for any type of exercise, it is helpful to perform the motion parallel with the floor. Motions that are perpendicular to the floor and moving toward the floor are being aided by gravity.

Initial or starting position may have a profound influence on the safety and merit of the flexibility exercise. Starting positions should be evaluated to determine if structures are being inappropriately stretched. A good example of an inappropriate starting position is the exercise called the "hurdler's stretch." This starting position places undue stress on the medial collateral ligaments by stretching excessively the inside of the knee (see figure 4.14).

The initial position of an exercise may have a particular adverse reaction for persons with certain disabilities. Care must be taken to insure that persons with hyperreflexive muscles are not placed in a starting position that will activate muscle groups. For example, a student with CP may be placed in excessive dorsiflexion at the ankle. This position may cause the calf muscle to contract. Another consideration when helping persons with abnormal reflex activity involves the positioning of the teacher or helper. Eye contact should be at a level position so the student

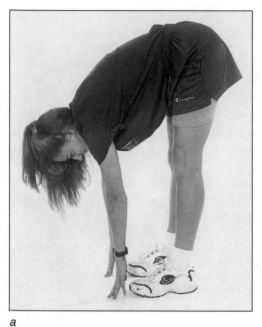
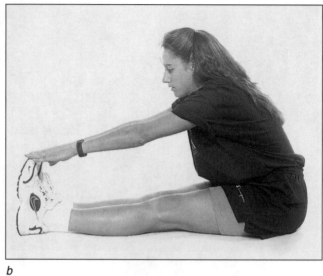

Figure 4.13a–b Toe-touch: (*a*) standing and (*b*) sitting

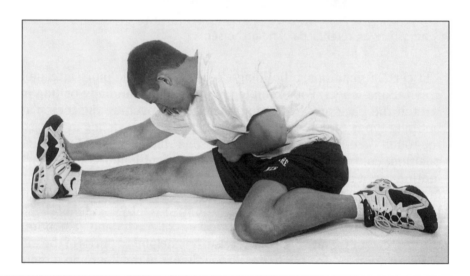

Figure 4.14 Hurdler's stretch (contraindicated)

does not have to hyperextend the neck. If a person is in a sitting position and has to look up at the teacher, the extension position of the neck can cause an extension reaction of various muscle groups, which can negate the benefits of various types of flexibility exercises. Extension of the spine may cause a student to slide down from the erect sitting position. Also, if the teacher is trying to have the student first extend and then flex the elbow, the extension position will be dominant.

Muscle Imbalance

A problem associated with flexibility/ROM is imbalance in strength or ROM between agonistic and antagonistic muscle groups. There are several reasons for the condition of muscle imbalance. One cause for muscle imbalance is the way one muscle group is used more than another in ADLs and sporting activities. For example, as one reads a book while sitting at a desk, there is a tendency to be somewhat round-shouldered. Over a period of time the anterior chest muscles (pectoralis major and minor) will adjust to this shorter position. Other muscles, such as rhomboids major and minor, tend to be elongated over a period of time. The net result is that the anterior chest muscles will feel tight when the arms are abducted and extended. To achieve appropriate balance the anterior chest muscles will need to be subjected to flexibility exercises, and upper back muscles (rhomboids) will need to be strengthened.

Muscle imbalance often results from frequent involvement in certain physical activities. Individuals involved in striking motions, such as in softball and wheelchair tennis, may have a muscle imbalance between shoulder internal and external rotators. These individuals may have tight internal rotators and benefit from flexibility exercises. The external shoulder rotators may benefit from additional strength development exercises. Although greater emphasis may be placed on flexibility exercises for numerous muscle groups, all muscle groups should be involved in both strength and flexibility exercise programs. Imbalance may result from ADLs. A student sitting in a wheelchair and using a computer keyboard may develop round shoulders. Certain anterior chest muscles are tight. If this student sits in a wheelchair over long periods of time and has an above-knee amputation, the sitting position may cause the hip flexors to shorten. Thus, there is an imbalance in length of the hip flexors in relation to the hip extensors.

Another reason for muscle imbalance may be the neuromuscular problems associated with a kind of disability. With upper motor neuron lesions (UMNLs), muscle groups will be in a state of partial or full contraction for extended periods of time. The net effect is that muscle groups manifest exceptional muscle tone and varying degrees of strength. The antagonistic muscles, however, are comparably weaker and in a somewhat elongated position. An example of this situation is the exceptional muscle tone and contracted state of flexor, abductor, and internal rotator muscles of persons with spastic CP. Wrist flexors are in a shortened, contracted, tight position. The wrist extensors are in an elongated position and are not equal in strength to the flexors. Working on ROM for wrist extension and dealing with this imbalance would involve some type of ROM or flexibility exercise for the wrist flexors and strength development for the wrist extensors.

Adjustments for Spasticity

With certain types of disabilities, the challenge of developing various facets of physical fitness is exacerbated by the presence of spasticity. Damage to the central nervous system, such as the cerebral cortex with spastic CP or in other types of brain trauma, results in hyperactive reflexes and spasticity. Spasticity is a type of paralysis because it prevents movement.

Paralysis of any type necessitates the implementation of intervention strategies. This applies to the spastic type, which prevents movement, and to the flaccid type, which is characterized by no movement. In the case of spastic paralysis, ways must be devised to reduce the contracted state of muscle groups. If this state is reduced, then ROM exercises may be more effectively implemented.

A key factor for increasing ROM with spastic paralysis is to elongate the spastic muscle without activating the stretch reflex. A student with spastic CP has a type of flexion paralysis. A physical educator will want to work on extension movements. For example, if this is accomplished at the shoulder, the increase in ROM will enable the student to more effectively do ADLs. The operative word is *relaxation*. This may be accomplished by doing exercises in a warm swimming pool or aided by quiet handling of a student by the teacher. Some of the direct relaxation techniques discussed earlier would be applicable for spastic paralysis. Part of this approach may be to work on one joint or single-joint muscles. The process may then evolve to multiple joints and biarticular muscles.

Another factor deals with the positioning of the person. Certain postures or positions may elicit reflexive action. For example, students with UMNLs may still exhibit primitive reflexes, such as the asymmetrical tonic neck reflex. Students exhibiting this reflex turn their head to one side, particularly in a relaxed state, and extend the upper extremity on that side. Any attempt to work on elbow flexion will be counterproductive with the elicitation of this reflex. In this situation the head should be kept in a neutral position when working on ROM or flexibility.

Certain PNF exercises have potential application for persons with spasticity. Contract-relax and hold-relax are techniques used to deal with spasticity or neurological hypertonicity. The "hold" or "contract" phase of these techniques are applied to spastic muscles followed by the relax phase and subsequent elongation of the spastic muscle.

Coping With Contractures

Different disabilities—such as CP, certain congenital anomalies, amputations and SCIs—affect muscular and connective tissue in an adverse manner. Because of problems with the neuromuscular system, these types of tissue may alter the degree of motion in a joint. Spasticity, immobilization, paralysis, pain, and muscle imbalance may cause a shortening of muscle and connective tissue. A condition of fixed resistance to elongation of muscle because of a fibrous reaction of tissue associated with muscle and joints is referred to as a contracture.

Lack of motion and diminished physical activity is the precursor for contractures. The spasticity of a person with CP is often accompanied by contractures of the calf muscle, hip adductors, and elbow flexors. Immobilization of the shoulder may result in contractures of the joint affecting shoulder abductors and external rotators. With some individuals the severity of the contracture may necessitate surgery.

Contractures may also be the result of flaccid paralysis in which muscles are no longer able to cause movement at a joint because of neurological (polio myelitis) or muscular (muscular dystrophy) problems; this lack of movement results in joint contractures. Passive ROM exercises may prevent these contractures. Providing persons with disabilities with ROM exercises or activities may be included as a facet of a rehabilitation program. This may be applicable for both strength and ROM improvement; however, both are definitely facets of physical fitness. There will be times when the physical educator or adapted physical educator will be dealing with either rehabilitation and/or physical fitness enhancement situations when providing physical fitness activities for persons with disabilities.

Contraindicated Exercises

In this section characteristics of inappropriate exercises will be discussed. There are, however, some general situations where flexibility/ROM exercise would be considered inappropriate. If a person has joint swelling, edema, or joint infection, stretching exercises should not be conducted. If a student has any type of inflammatory disease and this condition seems to be getting worse, ROM exercise should not be done.

There are other conditions or situations where clearance should be obtained from a physician or physical therapist before having a student engage in a flexibility program. These include:

- individuals who have had surgery and exhibit extensive scarring and tissue adhesions;
- individuals with extreme spasticity and severe joint contractures;
- individuals with conditions relating to extreme mobility; and
- individuals with a history of joint subluxation, dislocation, or a condition of hypermobility, such as students with Down's syndrome.

As one develops a physical fitness program for any individual with or without a disability, the objective is to help improve their health status rather than to cause or exacerbate a condition. Certain commonly used flexibility exercises are questionable for persons without disabilities and contraindicated for individuals with disabilities. Inappropriate or contraindicated exercises share common characteristics. First, they tend to rely upon gravity to help in the stretching process. The danger with this type of exercise is the activation of the stretch reflex, which causes a contraction of the target muscle group rather than a relaxation of these muscles. As noted in an earlier section of this chapter the "toe-touch," which involves standing and touching the toes, is a flexibility exercise that for many persons with disabilities may cause musculotendinous problems rather than enhancing back and hamstring flexibility.

A second characteristic of a contraindicated flexibility exercise is the position or movement of the exercise, which places undue strain on various structures of the body. Again, an earlier section alluded to the "hurdler's exercise" (see figure 4.14). The initial position, which is assumed throughout the exercise, places undue strain on knee ligaments. While this type of strain will cause problems for any person, an exercise placing stress on these structures of persons with disabilities will increase the possibility of injury or joint damage. Particularly with persons who exhibit a disability, the exercise leader should initially analyze all positions and movements of any flexibility exercises to determine if the exercise will worsen the disability or create some other type of injury. If it is believed there is a possibility of undue stress on a structure or structures, the exercise should be eliminated from the exercise regimen. For example, "head rolls," in which a person rolls the head in a complete circle, are stressful to the upper spine (see figure 4.15). The rolling motion tends to cause excessive extension, which for a variety of orthopedic conditions may result in increased nerve pressure. Rather, have the person stretch neck muscles from side to side and then front to back. A student may control all the motions more easily and avoid excessive extension. The rolling motion may potentially cause problems with cervical vertebrae one and two.

There are situations where partner exercises may be contraindicated. A student engaging in partner stretching activities must be aware of exactly how much force should be applied. A student with a disability may not benefit from a peer tutor helping with flexibility exercises. The peer tutor may not have sufficient training in estimating the correct amount of force to apply. Also, there may be a tendency to apply excessive force because the peer tutor is not attending properly to the task at hand.

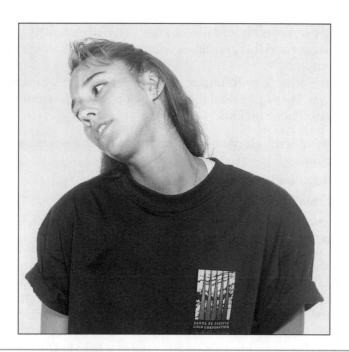

Figure 4.15 Head rolls (contraindicated)

Specific Exercises to Be Avoided

A sample of exercises will be described that fall into the category of contraindicated exercises. These exercises may rely excessively upon the effect of gravity, compromise body structures, or involve both of these characteristics.

As noted, "head rolls" place stress on spinal structures. Another exercise, the "yoga plow," where a person in a back lying position brings the feet up and over the head with the intent of stretching the back muscles, is contraindicated because it may develop a problem or injury to the back (see figure 4.16). Unfortunately, this position places excessive stress on the vertebral discs in the neck, which may cause a sprain or strain or may increase disc pressure.

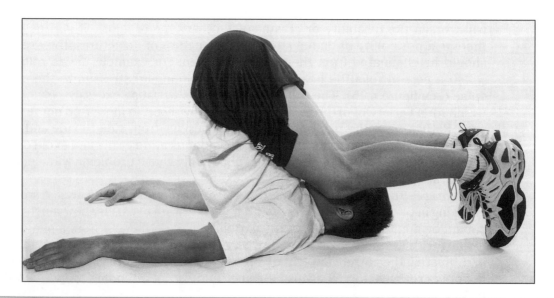

Figure 4.16 Yoga plow (contraindicated)

Another exercise, the "back bow," where a person is on his or her stomach and uses the hands to pull the feet and hyperextend the back, is also inappropriate (see figure 4.17). Again this position places excessive stress on the vertebrae in the thoracic and lumbar areas.

The common exercise of "trunk circling" may cause several problems. In this exercise, a person bends forward at the waist, bends laterally to one side, extends the back, and finally bends laterally to the other side of the body. First, the hyperextended position assumed during part of this exercise reinforces a lordotic position. The flexed position with the knees locked increases intervertebral disc pressure in the lumbar region.

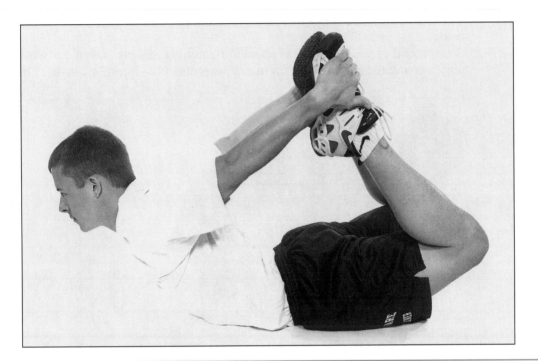

Figure 4.17 Back bow (contraindicated)

The "hip-back stretcher" is an exercise that may cause more harm than good. A person assumes a kneeling position, hyperextends the back, and grasps the ankles. This exercise is intended to stretch the hip flexor. Again, hyperextension of the spine will place excessive stress on the vertebral discs and should not be an exercise of choice. Another exercise, if done incorrectly, may cause musculotendonous problems. This is the "calf stretching" exercise. In this exercise, a person stands a selected distance from a wall and then leans and touches the wall. If too far away from the wall or forcefully pushing and bobbing, the activation of the stretch reflex may cause deleterious effects on the calf muscle. If a person is trying to stretch the calf muscles and these muscles are reflexively contracting, the net result may be a tearing of muscle tissue.

Recommended Stretching Movements

Stretching exercises may be addressed from two approaches. One approach is called the agonist (target)-antagonist method, which requires an understanding of motion or motions of the antagonistic muscle. If a person understands the relationship between the agonist and antagonist muscles and their respective motions, then a flexibility exercise may be simplistically devised by elongating the target muscle by means of activating the antagonist muscle. For example, if the target muscle is the biceps, then concentric (shorter) contractions of the triceps will stretch the biceps. This elongation or stretch of the biceps may be done as a passive exercise or an active exercise. For students with CP, extension motions at the elbow may be quite beneficial. The stretching of the biceps and contraction of the triceps may be part of a PNF protocol. For example, to implement the hold-relax technique, the arm would be passively extended until the bicep was in a stretched position. From this extended position an isometric contraction of the biceps would be done with a partner providing the appropriate resistance. Relaxation of the biceps would follow the isometric contraction, and the partner or teacher would then extend the elbow, placing the biceps again into an elongated position.

The second approach is to use specific stretching exercises, some of which have their own names, such as the "mad cat" exercise (see figure 4.18a–b). This exer-

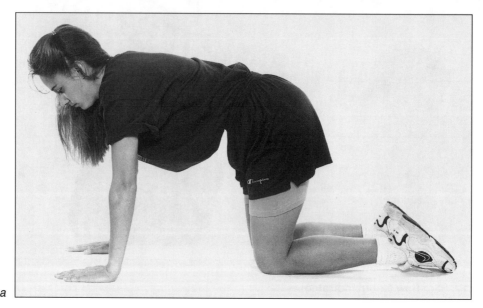

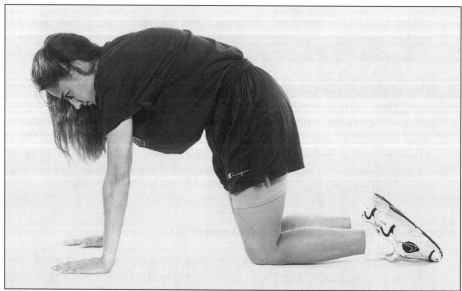

Figure 4.18a–b Mad cat exercise: (*a*) rest position and (*b*) stretching back muscles

cise is done by getting down on all fours and arching the back like a frightened or mad cat. The purpose of this exercise is to stretch the back muscles. The stretching motion is against gravity. Many of these specifically named exercises are done using a static stretching technique.

While an entire book could be devoted to these exercises, a brief overview will be provided. This overview will address each major joint in the body and in certain cases will be the exercise of choice rather than the contraindicated exercise mentioned in the previous section.

Neck

To help develop flexibility of neck muscles, the "basic four" exercise may be done. The student should first flex and then extend the neck. This is followed by lateral flexion to the right and then to the left. The student should avoid degrees of hypermotion, such as hyperextension. These movements should be substituted for the "head rolls" exercise.

Shoulder

The shoulder involves six basic movements (flexion, extension, abduction, adduction, internal rotation, and external rotation) plus combination movements, such as horizontal adduction (flexion and adduction). Lying on his or her back, have the student abduct the arm to 90°, flex the elbow 90°, and externally rotate the arm. This exercise, called the "rotator," will stretch shoulder flexor and internal

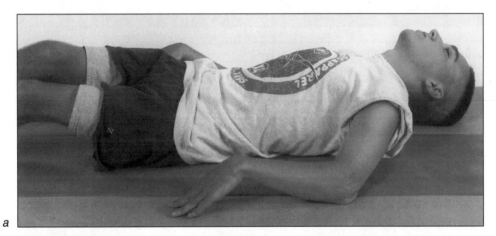

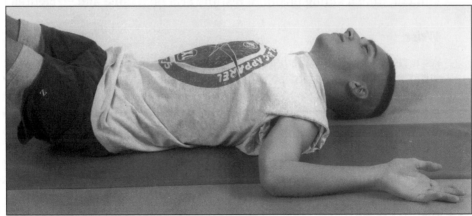

Figure 4.19a–b Rotation of the shoulder: (*a*) internal rotation and (*b*) external rotation

rotator muscles (see figure 4.19a–b). Rotating from external rotation to internal rotation will stretch the external rotators. Using the same starting position, which is shoulder abduction to 90° and elbow fixed at 90°, have the student horizontally adduct the arm so the hand touches the other shoulder. This exercise will stretch shoulder extensors and some abductors (see figure 4.20).

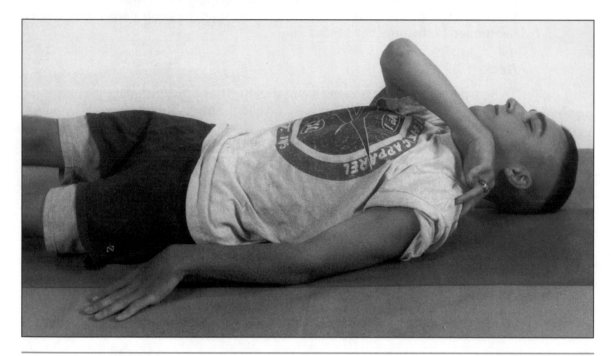

Figure 4.20 Shoulder horizontal adduction

Shoulder and Elbow

The modified Apley test used for flexibility evaluation in the BPFT may also be used as an exercise to stretch elbow and shoulder extensors. In this test, the participant attempts to touch the mouth, top of the head, and, if possible, the superior angle of the opposite scapula. If the back of the hand touches the back, the supinator of the elbow will also be stretched. In a sitting or standing position have the student try to touch the ceiling. This will stretch elbow flexors. If there is not enough strength to hold the arm in this flexed position at the shoulder, have the student, from a sitting position, rest the arm on a table and straighten it out.

Wrist

As a teacher tries to develop flexibility/ROM of the student's upper extremity, wrist motion should not be neglected. An exercise to work on wrist ROM is the "carpal" exercise. Have the student place the forearm on a table or on his or her lap with the arm in a pronated position, and bring the back of the hand toward the body (see figure 4.21a). This may be done with the aid of the other hand. This exercise will stretch the wrist flexors. A variation of this exercise is to place the palm on the table and raise (extend) the hand toward the ceiling. Have the student change from a pronated to a supinated position and repeat the exercise. In this position the wrist extensors will be stretched as the student flexes the wrist (see figure 4.21b).

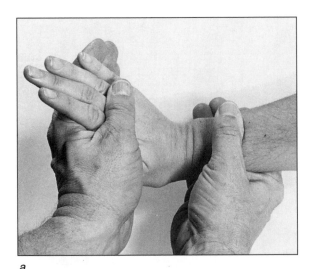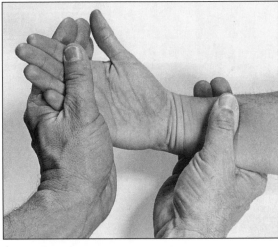

a   b

Figure 4.21a–b Developing wrist extension flexibility by (*a*) stretching wrist flexors and (*b*) stretching wrist extensors

Back

Two exercises called the "back flattener" and "knee pull" are recommended to stretch the back. A student assumes a supine position, places the hands in the small of the back, and tries to squeeze the hands with the back. This exercise will stretch the lumbar portion of the back (see figure 4.22). Still on the back, the student grabs the knees and slowly brings them to the chest. This movement may be repeated several times (see figure 4.23). This exercise is much better than toe-touches for stretching back muscles, since one is less likely to bounce or bob because there is very little gravitational assistance.

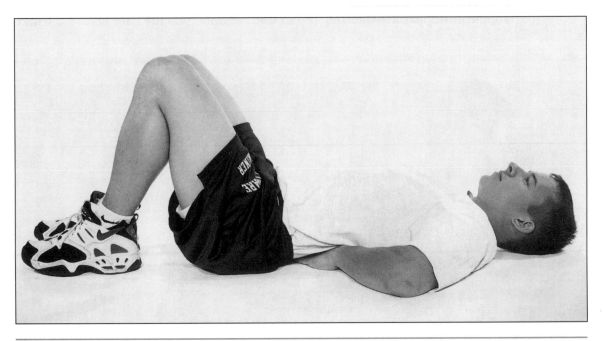

Figure 4.22 Stretching back muscles

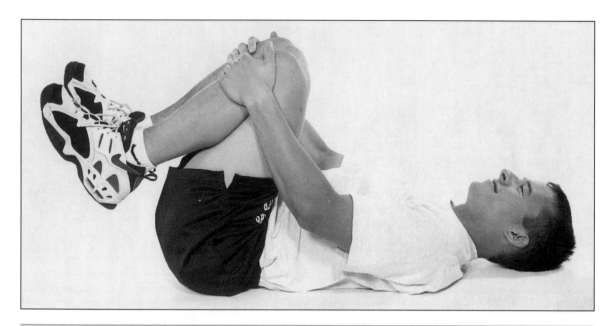

Figure 4.23 Knees to chest exercise

Hip

Two exercises are recommended for stretching hip muscles. The first exercise, called the "extensor stretch," is started by having the student sit on the edge of a bed or bench with one leg extended. With the back kept straight, the student bends from the hips and grasps the ankle or lower leg. This exercise does not put strain on the collateral ligaments of the knees as does the hurdler's stretch. The second exercise is the "Ober exercise." In a standing position, the student brings one leg across the body and places the foot outside the other foot. This position will stretch the hip abductors. A variation of this exercise may be done in the supine position. Have the student flex one knee and pull the knee across the mid-

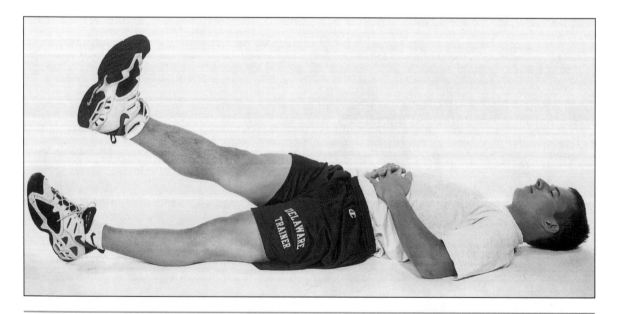

Figure 4.24 Abductor stretch with knee extended

line (see figure 4.24). Then have the student straighten the knee that has been bent. This exercise will stretch the abductors and hip extensors.

Knee

Exercises designed to stretch knee flexors generally involve hip extensors because the knee flexors are biarticular muscles (hip and knee joints). A very simple exercise to stretch a knee flexor is to sit in an L position with the knees in an extended position. However, for certain persons with disabilities, this may be too stressful. An alternative exercise is to have the person assume a side-lying position. The individual attempts to straighten the knees within a certain comfort zone. The "extensor stretch" described in the previous paragraph also stretches knee flexors and is not very stressful to the vertebrae.

Ankle and Calf

An important area to stretch is the calf muscles, which provide ankle motion. The "toe-to-nose" exercise will help to establish good ROM at the ankle (figure 4.25). While sitting on the floor, the student loops a towel around the feet and gradually pulls the towel bringing the toes toward the nose (Grady and Saxena, 1991). This is a much better exercise than standing near a wall and lunging forward to stretch the plantar flexors (calf plus other foot muscles). In the interest of full ROM at the ankle, the anterior ankle muscles (dorsiflexors) should be stretched. The "heel-toe pull" can help establish the desired degrees of plantar flexion. In a sitting position with one leg crossed, the student grasps the toes with one hand and the heel with the other hand and pulls the toes away from the knee. This exercise will stretch the dorsiflexors.

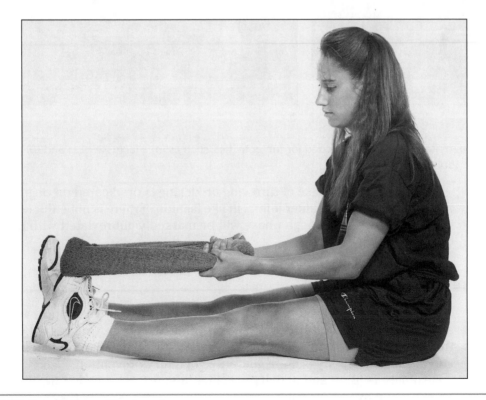

Figure 4.25 Dorsiflexion with a towel

VALUE OF FLEXIBILITY IN A PHYSICAL FITNESS PROGRAM

A certain amount of flexibility is needed to efficiently and effectively execute ADLs and sport-related movements. ADLs require varying amounts of ROM and flexibility. For a student with lower extremity limitations, the use of crutches is important for walking. Limited flexion or extension at the shoulders will reduce the efficiency of this person's gait. When a person kicks a soccer ball or throws a softball, a certain amount of flexibility at the hip or shoulder is needed for the preparatory and execution phases of both skills. To throw a ball a person must have sufficient external rotation during the preparatory phase to bring the arm into the windup or cocking phase (see figure 4.26a–b). If there is not sufficient movement during this phase "to reach back to throw," very little force may be applied to the ball during the execution phase.

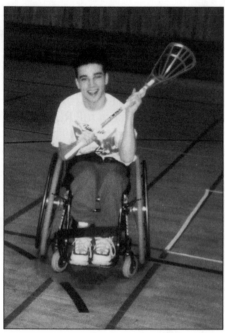

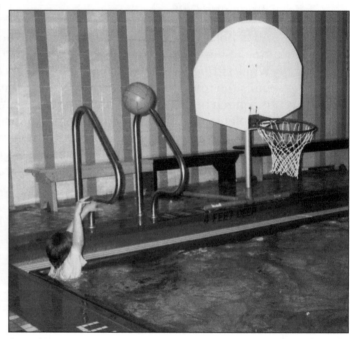

a

b

Figure 4.26a–b Range of motion needed for fun activities, such as (*a*) a lacrosse pass and (*b*) a basketball throw in the pool

This preparatory phase of throwing or kicking is predicated on degrees of flexibility in the hip or shoulder joints. In like fashion, if there is not sufficient internal rotation, the follow-through phase will be markedly abbreviated with dire consequences to skill execution.

Prevention of Injury

There is enough evidence to establish a relationship between optimal flexibility and the reduction of rate, degree, and duration of injuries. One of the key terms in the first sentence is *optimal level of flexibility*. More flexibility is not always better, and maximal flexibility is not a guarantee of injury prevention.

Flexibility is joint- and activity-specific. In sport, the needed flexibility of the hamstrings may vary. For the hurdler, increased extensibility may be needed to a much greater extent than for a mile runner. The needed flexibility of the shoulder for a gymnast is different than that of a football lineman. The same concept applies to students with disabilities. A student with CP may need limited external rotation to participate in an adapted bowling situation but will need more external rotation to comb the hair at the back of the head.

Condition Enhancement

Certain types of flexibility exercises may help ameliorate a by-product of physical fitness activities. During the early stages of a fitness or activity program, a participant may experience muscle soreness. Slow, static stretching exercises have been found to alleviate discomfort of sore muscles. Part of the explanation for this effect is based upon de Vries' (1966) spasm theory. Soreness in muscles is in part due to muscle spasm or a slight contraction of muscle. Static stretching elongates muscle and reduces electrical activity with accompanying reduction in muscle discomfort.

Reduction of muscle activity may also be related to another benefit of stretching. There are various types and kinds of stress—physical, mental, and emotional. There is evidence that physical activity assists in stress reduction or stress management (Morgan and Horstman, 1976). For many individuals stress is manifested in muscle twitching and tightness. Flexibility exercises may help to reduce this tightness.

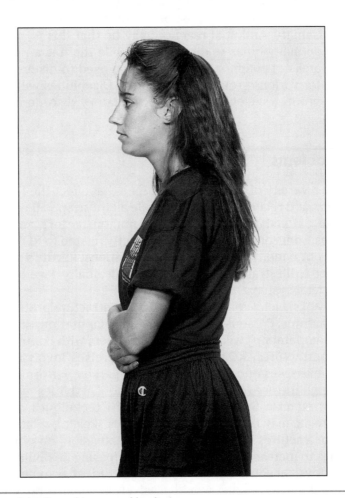

Figure 4.27 Anterior pelvic tilt and increased lordosis

Flexibility enhancement provides another benefit to total body fitness, namely, body symmetry. Overdevelopment or constant use of selected muscle groups may lead to asymmetrical body development. For example, individuals using crutches and a swing-through gait pattern may excessively use shoulder flexor muscles. Upper chest and shoulder muscles may become overly developed. The net result may be the development of rounded shoulders. Stretching these overdeveloped muscles will help to reestablish chest-back symmetry. For total chest-back symmetry, the pectoral muscles should be stretched or elongated and the back muscles, such as trapezius and rhomboids, should be strengthened.

Another example of body symmetry is the relationship between abdominal and erector spinal muscles. If the erector spinal muscles are too tight, an increase in the lumbar curve will occur because the pelvis will be anteriorly titled (see figure 4.27). If the erector spinal muscles have sufficient flexibility and the abdominal muscles are well developed, more of a posterior pelvic tilt will be assumed in the standing position with less lordotic curve. Symmetry of the body involves flexibility with agonistic muscles and an appropriate amount of strength development in other muscles.

FLEXIBILITY AND SPECIFIC TYPES OF DISABILITIES

As a person develops a flexibility program for individuals with disabilities, considerations and adaptations must be oriented toward the specific characteristics of each disability. An initial reaction may be that this is an impossible task, for there are so many types of disabilities. While there is a plethora of disabilities, there are areas of commonality that can be used to discuss the development of flexibility for various groups of disabilities. Disabilities will be classified into the following groups: skeletal problems, circulatory disorders, and neuromuscular disorders.

Skeletal Problems

There are a variety of disabling conditions that affect the functioning of the skeletal system and related structures. While all these specific conditions would constitute an extensive list, there are common factors among skeletal-related disabilities. Some of these factors are directly related to ROM and flexibility development. Four conditions—arthritis, amputations, Perthe's disease, and obesity—will be used to illustrate concepts related to flexibility development and disabilities of the skeletal system.

A variety of skeletal conditions will have contracture problems, particularly flexion contractures. Persons with arthritis and amputations (i.e., the joint above the site of an amputation) will often have a problem with contractures. In the case of flexion contractures, ROM or flexibility exercises involving extension motions would be exercises of choice. Prior to the person performing, the application of heat through the use of heated swimming pool activities may enhance the execution of the exercise. Static stretching and PNF techniques, such as hold-relax and contract-relax, may be used to deal with this skeletal, related problem. Since hip flexion contractures prevent optimal hip extension, an objective of a flexibility program is to increase hip extension by increasing flexibility/ROM of the hip flexors. The physical educator could have the student assume a prone position on a bench or table. The teacher would passively extend the hip until resistance is felt. Care should be taken by the teacher to make sure the motion is at the hip and that there is no substituted motion involving back extension. The student then initiates hip flexion, with the teacher applying resistance as this motion is performed. This sequence would be repeated at least three times with the teacher initiating the sequence with passive hip extension. The teacher has involved this student in the PNF technique of contract-relax. Other physical activities may also be used to improve flexibility/ROM. Having students throw some variety of Nerf ball emphasizes extension motions. Aquatic activities, which emphasize hip adduction types of movement, will benefit students who are recovering from Perthe's disease.

Muscle imbalances may contribute to ROM and flexibility problems in persons with skeletal disabilities. Imbalances may exist at one or more sites. If muscles are tight or extremely well developed, then strength development of the antagonistic muscles will help develop total ROM.

Many skeletal-related disabilities manifest muscle contractures or a tightness of muscle groups. Persons with arthritis, amputations of the lower extremity, and Perthe's disease often have hip flexion contractures. Persons with arthritis also have tight hip adductors, whereas children with Perthe's disease have tight hip abductors. The goal of a flexibility program with any type of contracture or tightness is to increase the ROM of the restricted musculature and to develop the strength of the contralateral muscles. For example, the student recovering from Perthe's disease could be instructed to do the "Ober exercise" to stretch tight hip abductors.

Another factor to consider in regard to skeletal disabilities is the development of an adaptive posture. For example, a student with an above-knee amputation may develop flexion contractures of the hip. In a standing position the flexed hip position results in an increase in lordosis and low-back pain or discomfort. Stretching of the hip flexors and erector spinal muscles will help to counter this lordotic condition. Developing the strength of contralateral muscles, the abdominal and hip extensors, should also be a part of a person's flexibility program.

With any type of flexibility or ROM program, one must only stretch an affected joint to the point of pain. There are times that physical therapists may work on ROM, and pain or discomfort is experienced by the patient. In a fitness program, pain or discomfort of this type is not considered appropriate and beyond the parameters of a physical fitness program. By using the various approaches described in this chapter, a teacher can stretch or "overstretch" without causing pain.

Circulatory Disorders

Circulatory disorders and diseases are often not associated with flexibility or ROM deficiencies. There are two factors that a professional must address when developing a physical fitness program for persons with circulatory problems. The first factor, which is applicable to all circulatory problems, is the intensity level of exercises, including flexibility and ROM exercises.

The second factor is the accompanying symptoms associated with a certain disorder or disease. For illustrative purposes three conditions will be addressed: rheumatic heart disease, diabetes, and stroke (cardiovascular accidents).

A key factor related to persons with rheumatic heart disease is the intensity level of all activities, including flexibility exercises. The extent of heart damage and recovery are factors that will guide the physician's recommendation regarding physical activity selection and intensity level. Also, the intensity of physical activities is addressed in chapter 2. For many students, residual effects are minimal, and most flexibility exercises will be appropriate activities. One precaution related to this entire category of disability is the use of isometric contractions.

Isometric exercises may place too much of a strain on the circulatory system. For example the PNF technique of hold-relax may not be the technique of choice. Rhythmic initiation, which starts with passive movements, progresses to active-assisted movement, active movements, and finally resisted isotonic movements may be more appropriate.

Intensity level for a person with diabetes must be viewed from a different perspective. A student with diabetes must consider three components in his/her life every day. They are food intake, insulin dosage, and activity level or intensity. The activity level, including physical fitness activities, is a factor that must be considered on a daily basis. For example, if one is performing several flexibility exercises on a certain day, this must be considered along with food intake and insulin dosage.

Individuals with diabetes may develop circulatory disorders, which may result in gangrene and amputation. With surgical amputations the joint above the site of amputation is a major concern regarding loss of ROM. For persons with amputations it is important to establish and maintain maximum flexibility/ROM of existing joints. Over a period of time a person may lose some ROM and flexibility. A well-developed physical fitness program will help to preclude any type of loss by maintaining the established ROM. For example, an individual with an above-the-knee amputation may over a period of time lose some hip extension ROM because the hip flexors become tight. This tightness will affect functionality, such as an efficient gait pattern.

For the person with a cardiovascular accident (CVA), one must consider the extent of involvement or damage and the level of exercise intensity that is compatible with this person's present circulatory status. One must consider the totality of the circulatory system and specific areas of the body that have been affected by this stroke. For the person with a CVA there will be neurological damage. Paralyses of parts or even a side of the body may be present. The unaffected portion or joints of the body should be kept at an appropriate level of fitness. Flexibility and ROM of these joints should be monitored carefully because the functionality of this person is predicated upon the fitness level of these joints. For parts of the body affected by a CVA, the physical educator will be dealing with a student with flaccid paralysis.

Neuromuscular Disorders

It is beyond the scope and purpose of this book to discuss each neurological problem and disability. There is a way to classify neurological disorders into dichotomous categories. One category includes persons with upper motor neuron lesions (UMNLs) and the other category includes persons with lower motor neuron lesions (LMNLs).

Individuals with UMNLs have such conditions as CP, head injury to the brain, SCIs and multiple sclerosis (MS). Several symptoms of UMNLs have direct relevance to ROM and flexibility. Hyperactive reflexes and spasticity accompany UMNL situations. To help a person with UMNLs, such as someone with CP, it is important to establish or maintain suitable ROM or flexibility with procedures that minimize the spastic state of the individual. Prolonged, low-tension stretching may be the protocol of choice. Contractures of certain muscle groups, such as flexors and adductors, will have to be minimized if increased ROM is to be established. This may be done by reducing the tension of the flexors and adductors through implementation of PNF techniques, use of relaxation measures, and with low-tension prolonged stretching procedures. Another approach is to strengthen the contralateral muscles of the student with CP, in this case focusing on the extensors and abductors. Activities that emphasize extension and abduction are quite helpful. For a young child with CP, riding a tricycle helps work on hip extensors. For a student in a wheelchair, propelling the chair with the feet, if possible, will work on functional extension movements. Aquatic activities, both exercises and swimming strokes that emphasize extension and abduction, would be most appropriate to help reach goals of a flexibility program.

Because the stretch reflex is hyperactive with persons with UMNLs, it is important to avoid ballistic or quick movement stretching techniques. Also, pressure on spastic muscles should be avoided because a reflexive contraction may ensue. Appropriate ROM activities in a heated swimming pool may help to counter the hyperactive nature of these muscles.

LMNLs present a different set of symptoms. A person with a peripheral nerve injury—such as traumatic SCI, polio, or spina bifida—exhibits muscle flaccidity. A lack of muscle tone or atrophy of this tissue characterizes this state of flaccidity. An accompanying condition is joint contractures because of diminished movement capacity. Exercises to prevent contractures include passive or active-assisted movement of the affected joints. The level of the SCI will determine the type of flexibility/ROM program. For a student with a high thoracic-level injury, both upper and lower extremities will exhibit flaccid paralysis, and passive ROM would be the type of exercise recommended. For the student with spina bifida and a level of lesion at lumbar vertebrae five, the lower extremity would have a certain amount of flaccid paralysis. The upper extremity, however, would exhibit no type of paralysis, and flexibility exercises for a nondisabled student would be used for this extremity.

One must keep in mind when working with these persons that areas and joints of the body may not have normal ROM because of surgical intervention. An individual with spina bifida may have had a part of the spine fused together. Flexibility exercises for the lower part of the back would be contraindicated. Individuals with LMNLs, such as those with SCI, will not have sensory input. If a person is moving part of the body devoid of sensory awareness, care must be taken to avoid undue stress on muscles, tendons, and ligaments. Care should be taken to avoid placing excessive weight on parts of the skeleton with this condition. Depending on the level of the lesion, bowel and bladder function may be affected, and it is important not to impair appliances used to assist excretory functions. Exercises involving the hip area may tangle up a tube to the collecting bag. For the physical educator, assistance and advice should be sought from the student's physician as well as other medical personnel regarding appropriate exercises and ways to execute them.

ANNOTATED RESOURCE LIST

WRITTEN RESOURCES

Adams, R.C., and McCubbin, J.A. (1991). Games, sports, and exercises for the physically disabled. Philadelphia: Lea & Febiger.

Provides a wide variety of games, sports, and exercises for persons with physical disabilities. They may be used as a means of improving strength, flexibility, endurance, aerobic capacity, and body composition.

American College of Sports Medicine (ACSM). (1997). Exercise management for persons with chronic diseases and disabilities. Champaign, IL: Human Kinetics.

Focuses on how to effectively manage exercise for someone with chronic disease or disability. The book includes 40 chapters categorized by disabilities, diseases, or conditions written by persons with clinical and research experience in exercise programming. Prominent in the book are suggestions for exercise testing and exercise programming.

Fleck, S., and Kraemer, W. (1997). Designing resistance training programs. Champaign, IL: Human Kinetics.

Presents physiological foundations, prescription methods, and training systems related to the use of resistance to develop strength and muscular endurance. In addition, the authors provide methods for training women, children, and seniors and methods for training athletes in specific sports. It includes excellent resources.

Goldberg, B. (Ed.). (1995). Sports and exercise for children with chronic health conditions. Champaign, IL: Human Kinetics.

Presents information on general issues related to sports, exercise, and chronic health conditions and subsequently provides specific information on these topics in chapters organized according to 20 disabilities and conditions. Chapters typically provide a brief description of disabilities or conditions, and they discuss exercise and sport programs in association with them.

Hesson, J. (1995). Weight training for life training. Englewood, CO: Morton.

Presents principles of resistance training to develop strength and muscular endurance and provides explanations of individual exercises. It provides resources and charts to help develop programs.

Jones, J.A. (1988). Training guide to cerebral palsy sports. Champaign, IL: Human Kinetics.

Focuses upon the development of athletes with physical disabilities for participation in a variety of sports (archery, riflery, swimming, boccia, bowling, cycling, soccer, handball, and track and field events). In regard to physical exercise, a strong chapter on weight training, including several exercises, is presented.

Miller, P. (Ed.). (1995). Fitness programming and physical disability. Champaign, IL: Human Kinetics.

This is an excellent edited book regarding the physical fitness of persons with disabilities. All chapters have relevance to the topic. Information in chapters includes the following:

- Basic principles of conditioning for the development of health-related physical fitness for persons with disabilities
- Guidelines for developing resistance training programs with general considerations for persons with disabilities
- Modifications for using stretch bands or tubing as a mode of exercise with persons with disabilities
- Ways of maintaining and developing flexibility, in general, and for persons with disabilities, in particular
- Exercises for the neck, shoulder, elbow, wrist, trunk, hip, knee, and ankle with modifications for persons with disabilities
- Intervention and emerging procedures associated with grand mal and petit mal seizures, ketoacidosis, hypoglycemia, autonomic dysreflexia, heat exhaustion, heat stroke, and postural and exercise hypotension
- Information relating to wheelchairs, exercising in a wheelchair, and transfers

Pangrazzi, R.P., and Corbin, C.B. (1994). Teaching strategies for improving youth fitness (2nd ed.). Reston, VA: AAHPERD.

This book was written to provide fitness ideas and activities to complement the Prudential *FITNESSGRAM*. Activities are suggested for developing aerobic capacity, body composition, muscular strength and endurance, and flexibility from the primary level through the secondary level. A small section is presented on modifying fitness programs and activities for individuals with unique needs.

Rimmer, J. (1994). Fitness and rehabilitation programs for special populations. Dubuque, IA: McGraw-Hill.

Presents exercise prescriptions and guidelines for a variety of special populations. Good ideas for physical activity are also given throughout the book. This book focuses on fitness and rehabilitation programs for persons with the following diseases/conditions: aging, arthritis, obesity, diabetes, asthma and other pulmonary diseases, spinal cord injury, and mental retardation.

Shephard, R.J. (1990). Fitness in special populations. Champaign, IL: Human Kinetics.

This is a comprehensive book covering a wide variety of topics. Topics of particular relevance to fitness training include responses to exercise and training, methods of fitness measurement, training programs, and practical issues in program design.

Shephard, R.J. (1994). Aerobic fitness and health. Champaign, IL: Human Kinetics.

Covers the interaction among physical activity, aerobic fitness, and health; the physiological determinants of aerobic fitness; current levels of physical activity and aerobic fitness; the potential for improving current levels of aerobic fitness; and the potential impact of aerobic fitness on the health of the exerciser.

Thomas, T. (1986). Muscular fitness through resistance training. Dubuque, IA: Eddie Bowers.

Discusses both principles and methods of strength and flexibility training. The focus is on adults. This book provides chapters on nutritional issues, training females, and how to use different resistance mechanisms.

Walsh, C.M, Hoy, D.J., and Holland, L.J. (1982). Flexibility exercises for the "wheelchair" user. Edmonton, AB: Research and Training Centre for the Physically Disabled. Faculty of Physical Education and Recreation.

This book is a helpful resource on flexibility exercises for the upper body and lower body of wheelchair users. The exercises have been designed so that they can be carried out anywhere. A few of the exercises require the assistance of a partner, but most can be performed independently.

Walsh, C.M., and Steadward, R.D. (1984). Muscular fitness exercises for the wheelchair user. Edmonton, AB: Research and Training Centre for the Physically Disabled, Department of Physical Education and Sport Studies.

Provides easy-to-follow exercises for the development of muscular strength, endurance, and power for the wheelchair user. Exercises recommended involve free weights, household items, and one's own body weight for resistance. Exercises and variations are presented for the trunk, shoulder, chest, upper back, arm, and wrist. Guidelines are presented in regard to sets, repetitions, and load.

AUDIOVISUAL RESOURCES

Aerobics for quadriplegia, Aerobics for cerebral palsy, Aerobics for paraplegia, Aerobics for amputees. (1995). Disabled Sports USA, 451 Hungerford Drive, Suite 100, Rockville, MD 20850. (Videotapes).

These four videotapes are a part of the Fitness for Everyone series developed by the National Handicapped Sports and Recreation Association (NHSRA). In these videotapes, instructors accompanied by youngsters and adults exercising in wheelchairs, demonstrate easy to progressively more demanding aerobic activities. Helpful hints for safe and effective exercising are also provided. Running time is 33 minutes for each videotape.

Get those arms moving. (1989). TheraCise, P.O. Box 9100, Unit #107, Newton, MA 02159. (Videotape).

This is a home exercise videotape specifically designed by an occupational therapist for individuals with a variety of disabilities of the upper extremity. Passive, active-assisted, and light active exercises are demonstrated by an adult. Exercises involving the fingers, wrist, elbow, and shoulder that may be used by children and adolescents are presented. Running time is approximately 20 minutes.

Keep fit while you sit. (N.d.). Slabo Productions, 1057 South Crescent Heights, Los Angeles, CA 90035. (Videotape).

Provides an aerobic workout for persons with physical challenges. In this videotape three youngsters with physical challenges (post-polio and cerebral palsy) follow an adult demonstrating warm-up, cool-down, and aerobic exercises while sitting. The exercise session is assisted by a physical therapist and is endorsed by the American Paralysis Association. Running time is approximately 40 minutes.

Strength and flexibility for individuals with all types of physical disabilities. Tape 2. (1995). National Handicapped Sports and Recreation Association, 451 Hungerford Drive, Suite 100, Rockville, MD 20850. (Videotape).

Presents dynamic isotonic strength exercises demonstrated by an instructor and followed by an individual with a disability. Exercises focus on the use of tubing for resistance. Running time is approximately 50 minutes.

Nancy's special workout for the "physically challenged." (N.d.). Capture Productions. 6441 Inkster Road, Suite 240, Bloomfield Hills, MI 48301. (Videotape).

This is a 45-minute workout videotape, which starts with a warm-up, moves to a vigorous cardiovascular workout, and ends with a cool-down period. Exercises for persons at a variety of fitness stages are performed while sitting. Target heart rates for individuals at various ages and specific exercises for persons with hemiplegia are recommended.

REFERENCES

CHAPTER 1

American Alliance for Health, Physical Education, Recreation and Dance (AAHPERD). (1980). Health related physical fitness test manual. Washington, DC: AAHPERD.

American College of Sports Medicine (ACSM). (1995). ACSM's guidelines for exercise testing and preparation (5th ed.). Baltimore: Williams & Wilkins.

Blair, S.N. (1993). 1993 C.H. McCloy Research Lecture. Physical activity, physical fitness, and health. Research Quarterly for Exercise and Sport, *64*, 365-376.

Bouchard, C., and Shephard, R.J. (1994). Physical activity, fitness, and health: The model and key concepts. In C. Bouchard, R.J. Shephard, and T. Stephens (Eds.), Physical activity, fitness, and health: International proceedings and consensus statement (pp. 77-86). Champaign, IL: Human Kinetics.

Bouchard, C., Shephard, R.J., and Stephens, T. (Eds.). (1994). Physical activity, fitness, and health: International proceedings and consensus statement. Champaign, IL: Human Kinetics.

Caspersen, E.J., Powell, K.E., and Christenson, G.M. (1985). Physical activity, exercise, and physical fitness: Definitions and distinctions for health-related research. Public Health Reports, *100* (2), 126-131.

Consensus Development Conference. (1995). Physical activity and cardiovascular health. Bethesda, MD: National Institutes of Health.

Cooper Institute for Aerobics Research (CIAR). (1992). The Prudential *FITNESSGRAM* test administration manual. Dallas, TX: CIAR.

Council for Physical Education for Children (COPEC). (n.d.). Physical activity for children: A statement of guidelines. National Association for Sport and Physical Education. Reston, VA: NASPE Publications.

Kraus, H., and Hirschland, R.P. (1954). Minimum muscular fitness tests in school children. Research Quarterly, *25* (2), 178-188.

Lockette, K.F., and Keyes, A.M. (1994). Conditioning with physical disability. Champaign, IL: Human Kinetics.

Paffenbarger, R.S., Jr., and Lee, I-M. (1996). Physical activity and fitness for health and longevity. Research Quarterly for Exercise and Sport, *67*, Supplement to No. 3.

Pangrazzi, R.P., and Corbin, C.B. (1994). Teaching strategies for improving youth fitness. Reston, VA: The American Alliance for Health, Physical Education, Recreation and Dance.

Pangrazzi, R.P., Corbin, C.B., and Welk, G.J. (1996). Physical activity for children and youth. Journal of Physical Education, Recreation, and Dance, *67* (4), 38-43.

Pate, R.R. (1988). The evolving definition of fitness. Quest, *40*, 174-178.

Pate, R.R., Pratt, M., Blair, S.N., Haskell, W.L., Macera, C.A., Bouchard, C., Buchner, D., Ettinger, W., Heath, G.W., King, A.C., Kriska, A., Leon, A.S., Marcus, B.H., Morris, J., Paffenbarger, R.S., Patrick, K., Pollack, M.L., Rippe, J.M., Sallis, J., and Wilmore, J.H. (1995). Physical activity and public health. Journal of the American Medical Association, *273* (5), 402-407.

President's Council on Physical Fitness and Sports. (1996). Surgeon General's report on physical activity and health. Physical Activity and Fitness Research Digest, *2* (6), 1-8.

U.S. Department of Health and Human Services. (1996). Physical activity and health: A report of the Surgeon General. Atlanta, GA: U.S. Department of Health and Human Services, Center for Disease Control and Prevention, National Center for Chronic Disease Prevention and Health Prevention.

Winnick, J.P., and Short, F.X. (1999). The Brockport physical fitness test manual. Champaign, IL: Human Kinetics.

CHAPTER 2

American College of Sports Medicine (ACSM). (1995). ACSM's guidelines for exercise testing and prescription (5th ed.). Baltimore: Williams & Wilkins.

American College of Sports Medicine (ACSM). (1998). The recommended quantity and quality of exercise for developing and maintaining cardiorespiratory and muscular fitness, and flexibility in healthy adults. Medicine and Science in Sports and Exercise, *30* (6), 975-991.

Borg, G.A. (1998). Borg's perceived exertion and pain scales. Champaign, IL: Human Kinetics.

Borg, G.A. (1982). Psychological bases of perceived exertion. Medicine and Science in Sports and Exercise, *14,* 377-382.

Bouchard, C., and Shephard, R.J. (1994). Physical activity, fitness, and health: The model and key concepts. In C. Bouchard, R.J. Shephard, and T. Stephens (Eds.), Physical activity, fitness, and health: International proceedings and consensus statement (pp. 77-86). Champaign, IL: Human Kinetics.

Corbin, C.B, and Pangrazzi, R.P. (1996). How much physical activity is enough? Journal of Physical Education, Recreation, and Dance, *67* (4), 33-37.

Council for Physical Education for Children (COPEC). (n.d.). Physical activity for children: A statement of guidelines. National Association for Sport and Physical Education. Reston, VA: NASPE Publications.

Cureton, K.J. (1994). Aerobic capacity. In J.R. Morrow, H.B. Falls, and H.W. Kohl (Eds.), The Prudential *FITNESSGRAM* technical reference manual (pp. 33-55). Dallas, TX: The Cooper Institute for Aerobics Research.

Fernhall, B. (1997). Mental retardation. In ACSM (Ed.), Exercise management for persons with chronic diseases and disabilities: Champaign, IL: Human Kinetics.

Figoni. S.F. (1995). Physiology of aerobic exercise. In P. Miller (Ed.), Fitness programming and physical disability. Champaign, IL: Human Kinetics.

Heath, G.W., and Fentem, P.H. (1997). Physical activity among persons with disabilities—A public health perspective. Exercise and Sport Sciences Reviews, *25,* 195-234.

Ike, R.W., Lampman, R.M., and Castor, C.W. (1989). Arthritis and aerobic exercise: A review. Physician and Sports Medicine, *17* (2), 129-138.

Miller, P. (1995). Fitness programming and physical disability. Champaign, IL: Human Kinetics.

Pangrazzi, R., Corbin, C., and Welk, G. (1996). Physical activity for children and youth. Journal of Physical Education, Recreation, and Dance, *67* (4), 38-43.

Pate, R.R. (1995). Physical activity and health: Dose-response issues. Research Quarterly for Exercise and Sport, *66* (4), 313-317.

Pate, R.R., Pratt, M., Blair, S., Haskell, W., Macera, C., Bouchard, C., et al. (1995). Physical activity and public health: A recommendation for the Centers of Disease Control and Prevention and the American College of Sports Medicine, Journal of the American Medical Association, *273* (5), 402-407.

Rarick, G.L., Dobbins, D.A., and Broadhead, G.D. (1976). The motor domain and its correlates in educationally handicapped children. Upper Saddle River, NJ: Prentice Hall.

Rarick, G.L., and McQuillan, J.P. (1977). The factor structure of motor abilities of trainable mentally retarded children: Implications for curriculum development (Project No. H233544). Berkeley, CA: University of California, Department of Physical Education.

Rimmer, J. (1994). Fitness and rehabilitation programs for special populations. Dubuque, IA: McGraw-Hill.

Shephard, R.J. (1994). Aerobics fitness and health. Champaign, IL: Human Kinetics.

U.S. Department of Health and Human Services. (1996). Physical activity and health: A report of the Surgeon General, Atlanta, GA: U.S. Department of Health and Human Services, Centers for Disease Control and Prevention, National Center for Chronic Disease Prevention and Health Promotion.

Winnick, J.P., and Short, F.X. (1982). The physical fitness of sensory and orthopedically impaired youth. Project UNIQUE final report. Brockport, NY: State University of New York, College at Brockport (ERIC ED 240764).

Winnick, J.P., and Short, F.X. (1999). The Brockport physical fitness test manual. Champaign, IL: Human Kinetics.

CHAPTER 3

American College of Sports Medicine (ACSM). (1998). The recommended quantity and quality of exercise for developing and maintaining cardiorespiratory and muscular fitness, and flexibility in healthy adults. Medicine and Science in Sports and Exercise, *30* (6), 975-991.

American College of Sports Medicine (ACSM). (1995). ACSM's guidelines for exercise testing and prescription. Baltimore: Williams & Wilkins.

American Heart Association (AHA). (1992). Medical/scientific statement on exercise: Benefits and recommendations for physical activity for all Americans. Circulation, *85,* 2726-2730.

Council for Physical Education for Children (COPEC). (n.d.). Physical activity for children: A statement of guidelines. Reston, VA: NASPE Publications.

Davis, W., and Kelso, S. (1982). Analysis of "invariant characteristics" in motor control of Down's syndrome and normal subjects. Journal of Motor Development, *14*, 194-212.

Figoni, S., Lockette, K., and Surburg, P. (1995). Exercise prescription: Adapting principles of conditioning. In P. Miller (Ed.), Fitness programming and physical disability (pp. 65-78). Champaign, IL: Human Kinetics.

Fleck, S., and Kraemer, W. (1988). Resistance training: Physiological responses and adaptations. The Physician and Sports Medicine, *16* (4), 108-124.

Fleck, S., and Kraemer, W. (1997). Designing resistance training programs. Champaign, IL: Human Kinetics.

Howley, E.T., and Franks, B.D. (1997). Health fitness instructor's handbook. Champaign, IL: Human Kinetics.

Lockette, K. (1995). Resistance training: Program design. In P. Miller (Ed.), Fitness programming and physical disability (pp. 79-90). Champaign, IL: Human Kinetics.

Lockette, K., and Keyes, W. (1994). Conditioning with physical disability. Champaign, IL: Human Kinetics.

Miller, P. (1995). Skeletal muscle physiology and anaerobic exercise. In P. Miller (Ed.), Fitness programming and physical disability (pp. 35-50). Champaign, IL: Human Kinetics.

National Strength and Conditioning Association (NSCA). (1996). A position paper and literature review of youth resistance training. Colorado Springs: NSCA.

Pitetti, K., and Tan, D. (1991). Effects of a minimally supervised exercise program for mentally retarded adults. Medicine and Science in Sports and Exercise, *23*, 594-601.

President's Council on Physical Fitness and Sports (1996). Resistance Training for Health Research Digest, *2* (8), 1-6.

U. S. Department of Health and Human Services. (1996). Physical activity and health: A report of the Surgeon General. Atlanta, GA: U. S. Department of Health and Human Services. Centers for Disease Control and Prevention, National Center for Chronic Disease Prevention and Health Promotion.

Wilmore, J.H., and Costill, D.L. (1994). Physiology of sport and exercise. Champaign, IL: Human Kinetics.

Winnick, J.P., and Short, F.X. (1985). Physical fitness testing of the disabled. Champaign, IL: Human Kinetics.

CHAPTER 4

Alter, M.J. (1988). Science of stretching. Champaign, IL: Human Kinetics.

American Academy of Orthopaedic Surgeons. (1991). Athletic training and sports medicine (2nd ed.). Park Ridge, IL: OOHS.

American College of Sports Medicine (ACSM). (1995). ACSM's guidelines for exercise testing and prescription. Baltimore: Williams & Wilkins.

American College of Sports Medicine. (1998). The recommended quantity and quality of exercise for developing and maintaining cardiorespiratory and muscular fitness, and flexibility in healthy adults. Medicine and Science in Sports and Exercise, *30* (6), 975-991.

Anderson, B.S., and Burke, E.R. (1991). Scientific, medical, and practical aspects of stretching. Clinics in Sports Medicine, *10*, 63-68.

Bates, R.H. (1971). Flexibility training: The optimal time period to spend in a position of maximal stretch. Unpublished master's thesis, University of Alberta, Edmonton.

Benson, H. (1980). The relaxation response. New York: Avon Books.

Corbin, C.B., and Noble, L. (1980). Flexibility: A major component of physical fitness. The Journal of Physical Education and Recreation, *51*, 23-24, 57-60.

Council for Physical Education for Children (COPEC). (n.d.). Physical activity for children: A statement of guidelines. Reston, VA: NASPE Publications.

de Vries, H.A. (1966). Quantitative electromyographic investigation of the spasm theory of muscle pain. The American Journal of Physical Medicine, *45*, 119-134.

Grady, J.F., and Saxena, A. (1991). Effects of stretching the gastrocnemius. The Journal of Foot Surgery, *45*, 465-469.

Hardy, L. (1985). Improving active range of hip flexion. Research Quarterly for Exercise and Sport, *56*, 111-114.

Hollis, M. (1981). Practical exercise therapy. St. Louis: Blackwell Scientific.

Irrgang, J.J. (1994). Rehabilitation. In F. Fu and D.A. Stone (Eds.), Sports injuries (pp. 81-95). Baltimore: Williams & Wilkins.

Jacobson, E. (1938). Progressive relaxation. Chicago: University of Chicago Press.

Lasko, P.M., and Knopf, K.G. (1988). Adapted exercises for the disabled adult. Dubuque, IA: Eddie Bowers.

Lentell, G., Hetherington, T., Eagon, J., and Morgan, M. (1992). The use of thermal agents to influence the effectiveness of a low-load prolonged stretch. Journal of Orthopedic and Sports Therapy, *16*, 200-207.

Lockette, K., and Keyes, W. (1994). Conditioning with physical disability. Champaign, IL: Human Kinetics.

McArdle, W.D., Katch, F.L., Katch, B.L. (1994). Essentials of exercise physiology. Philadelphia: Lea & Febiger.

Markos, P. (1979). Ipsilateral and contralateral effects of proprioceptive neuromuscular facilitation techniques on hip motion and electromyographic activity. Physical Therapy, *59*, 1366-1373.

Massey, B.H., Johnson, W.R., and Kramer, G.F. (1961). Effect of warm-up exercise upon muscular performance using hypnosis to control the psychological variable. Research Quarterly, *32*, 63-71.

Morgan, W.P., and Horstman, D.H. (1976). Anxiety reduction following acute physical activity. Medicine and Science in Sports, *8*, 62.

Sapega, A.A., Quedenfeld, T.C., Moyer, R.A., and Butler, R.A. (1981). Biophysical factor in range-of-motion exercise. The Physician and Sports Medicine, *9*, 57-65.

Smith, C.A. (1991). The warm-up procedure: To stretch or not to stretch. A brief review. Journal of Orthopedic and Sports Physical Therapy, *19*, 12-17.

Surburg, P.R. (1981). Neuromuscular facilitation techniques in sports medicine. The Physician and Sports Medicine, *9*, 115-127.

Surburg, P.R. (1995). Flexibility training: Program design. In P. Miller (Ed.), Fitness programming and physical disability. Champaign, IL: Human Kinetics.

Surburg, P.R., and Schrader, J. (1997). Proprioceptive neuromuscular facilitation techniques in sports medicine—A reassessment. Journal of Athletic Training, 32, 34-39.

Voss, D.E., Ionta, M.K., and Myers, B.J. (1985). Proprioceptive neuromuscular facilitation. Philadelphia: Harper and Row.

Winnick, J., and Short, F. (1985). Physical fitness testing of the disabled. Champaign, IL: Human Kinetics.

Winnick, J.P., and Short, F.X. (1999). The Brockport physical fitness test manual. Champaign, IL: Human Kinetics.

INDEX

About the Authors

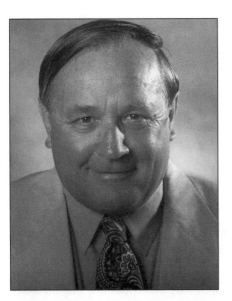

Joseph P. Winnick, EdD, is a distinguished service professor of physical education and sport at the State University of New York, College at Brockport. He received master's and doctoral degrees from Temple University. Dr. Winnick developed and implemented America's first master's degree professional preparation program in adapted physical education at Brockport in 1968 and since that time has secured funds from the U.S. Department of Education to support the program. He has been and continues to be involved in research related to the physical fitness of persons with disabilities. He is the editor of *Adapted Physical Education and Sport,* Second Edition (Human Kinetics, 1995). Dr. Winnick has received the G. Lawrence Rarick Research Award and the Hollis Fait Scholarly Contribution Award. In 1999, he received the Professional Recognition Award from the Adapted Physical Activity Council, American Alliance for Health, Physical Education, Recreation and Dance.

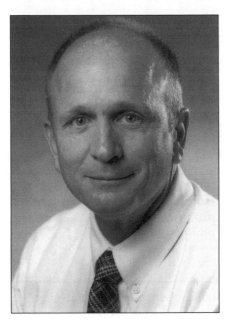

Francis X. Short, PED, is associate professor and chair of the Department of Physical Education and Sport at State University of New York, College at Brockport. Dr. Short has been involved with adapted physical education programs for the past 25 years. He has authored or coauthored numerous journal articles related to physical fitness and youngsters with disabilities. He is coauthor of *Physical Fitness Testing of the Disabled* (Human Kinetics, 1985) and author of "Physical Fitness," a chapter in *Adapted Physical Education and Sport*. He has served as project coordinator for three federally funded research projects pertaining to physical fitness and youngsters with disabilities. Dr. Short is a member of the American Alliance for Health, Physical Education, Recreation and Dance and the National Consortium on Physical Education and Recreation for Individuals with Disabilities.

RELATED RESOURCES

THE BROCKPORT PHYSICAL FITNESS TEST KIT

Joseph P. Winnick, EdD, and Francis X. Short, PED
1999 • CD-ROM for Windows • 3.5" disk for Windows

The test kit contains the three items below and the test manual, plus curl-up strips, skinfold calipers, and the PACER audiocassette and CD. The kit provides users with what they need to accurately assess fitness levels and to help students improve their fitness levels.

FITNESS CHALLENGE

Joseph P. Winnick, EdD, and Francis X. Short, PED
1999 • 3.5" diskettes

The companion software that makes using the Brockport Test much easier.

THE BROCKPORT PHYSICAL FITNESS TEST ADMINISTRATION VIDEO (APPROX 30-MINUTE VIDEOTAPE)

Joseph P. Winnick, EdD, and Francis X. Short, PED
1999 • VHS

Demonstrates clearly how to use the Brockport Physical Fitness Test for youths with physical and mental disabilities.

THE BROCKPORT PHYSICAL FITNESS TEST MANUAL

Joseph P. Winnick, EdD, and Francis X. Short, PED
1999 • Paperback • 168 pp

The manual presents all the test items that comprise the Brockport Test plus standards associated with desired levels of health-related physical fitness.

To request more information or to order, U.S. customers call 800-747-4457, e-mail us at **humank@hkusa.com**, or visit our website at **http://www.humankinetics.com/**. Persons outside the U.S. can contact us via our website or use the appropriate telephone number, postal address, or e-mail address shown in the front of this book.

THE AMERICAN FITNESS ALLIANCE

The Brockport Physical Fitness Test and Fitness Challenge software are offered through The American Fitness Alliance (AFA), a collaborative effort of AAHPERD, the Cooper Institute for Aerobics Research (CIAR), and Human Kinetics. AFA offers additional assessment resources, which can be combined with those listed above to create a complete health-related physical education program:

- The *FITNESSGRAM* test for evaluating students' physical fitness, developed by CIAR
- The *Physical Best Program*, which identifies the components of successful health-related physical education and provides the material needed to implement it in classes
- *FitSmart*, the first national test designed to assess high school students' knowledge of concepts and principles of physical fitness

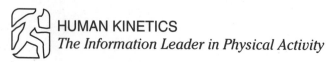 HUMAN KINETICS
The Information Leader in Physical Activity